bone-*loading*

**the new way
to prevent and
combat the
thinning bones of
osteoporosis**

bone-*loading*

the new way
to prevent and
combat the
thinning bones of
osteoporosis

ARIEL SIMKIN AND JUDITH AYALON

Foreword by HOWARD JACOBS MD, MRCP
Professor of Reproductive Endocrinology, Middlesex Hospital, London

PRION

First published in the United Kingdom in 1990 by
PRION, an imprint of Multimedia Books Limited,
32–34 Gordon House Road, London NW5 1LP

Editor Anne Cope
Photography Albi Zarfati
Photographic models Ora Chayoun, Boaz Rodansky
Design The Unknown Partnership
Production Arnon Orbach

British Library Cataloguing in Publication Data
Simkin, Ariel
    Bone-loading
    1. Man. Bones. Osteoporosis
    I. Title II. Judith Ayalon
    616.71

    ISBN 1 85375 037 8 hardback
    ISBN 1 85375 037 9 paperback

Typesetting and origination by Wyvern Typesetting Limited, UK
Printed in the United Kingdom by The Bath Press

contents

*Performing physical activities to preserve health –
such as playing with a ball, or wrestling, or pulling
the hands, or holding the breath – is considered by
fools a game of little value, and by the wise a good,
useful action.*

MOSES MAIMONIDES, philosopher, Talmudist and physician at
the court of Saladin (1135–1204 AD), in *Guide of the Perplexed*

AUTHORS' ACKNOWLEDGEMENT

Although the main subject of this book is the prevention of osteoporosis through bone-loading physical activity, we felt that readers would welcome information about other aspects of osteoporosis. Our sincere thanks go to various specialists and colleagues for their generous support and advice. Joseph Foldes MD of the Jerusalem Osteoporosis Center helped in the preparation of the sections on risk factors and medication; Professor Nathan Kaufmann, Head of the Department of Nutrition at the Hebrew University Medical School, read the sections on nutrition and osteoporosis and offered sensible suggestions; Isaac Leichter PhD of the Jerusalem Osteoporosis Center helped in the preparation of the section on the measurement of bone density.

In writing the main section of the book, the bone-loading exercise program, we were fortunate to have the advice and experience of Mrs Shlomit Raifmann-Levizky MPH. Last, but far from least, we would like to thank the lovely ladies who took part in the research which prompted this book and, we hope, a new and popular approach to the prevention and treatment of osteoporosis. They proved by their diligence and enthusiasm that the joys of physical exercise should not be confined to the young.

FOREWORD

At least three milestones can be identified in the history of the changing health of women. The first is the revolution in obstetrics, such that childbirth has become something most women anticipate with pleasure, rather than the serious challenge to survival it was before. It is salutary to recall that in 1566, when Mary Queen of Scots prepared for her first confinement, she and her court considered it prudent for her to write a will.

The second milestone concerns the control women have wrested from nature through the invention of birth control. In theory at least, the pivotal biological event of pregnancy can now be scheduled in time, place and number – and the scheduling is very largely in the individual woman's gift.

It is the third milestone that concerns the subject of this book. As a result of various improvements, largely social but to some extent medical too, men and women born in this century may with some confidence expect to live out their three score years and ten. For women this means that they will live some 20 to 30 years after the menopause. This demographically astounding fact – astounding because for women the medical implications of life beyond the menopause go much further than the effects of ageing – is only slowly being appreciated.

What are the biological implications of the menopause? Apart from the obvious loss of fertility and the distressing symptoms that can arise from the associated oestrogen deficiency, there is the hidden epidemic of osteoporosis, of brittle bones that fracture easily. This book contains much useful information on what causes a woman's skeleton to lose calcium after the menopause and so become a prey to oesteoporosis. But beyond the purely medical information and advice, Ariel Simkin and Judith Ayalon show women what they themselves can do to nurture their health and guard against the pain and immobility of osteoporotic fractures, fractures that might otherwise come at a time of life when we are least able to cope with them.

As a clinician much concerned with the hormonal details of the menopause and of its treatment, I welcome this book because it is based on sound physiological principles. Moreover, since few therapeutic endeavours are totally free of side effects (except, of course, for stopping smoking – which in addition to all of its well known benefits also eliminates one of the risk factors for osteoporosis), most clinicians welcome complementary treatments which permit therapeutic effects to be obtained with lower doses of drugs. Thus while I see the programme of exercises described herein as appropriate for most women who are concerned to prevent osteoporosis, I do not see it as an alternative to hormone treatment, particularly in women in whom oestrogen deficiency is evident. Clearly both are appropriate. I hope this book will help us all develop a more holistic approach to osteoporosis than has hitherto been the case.

Howard Jacobs MD, MRCP
Middlesex Hospital, London

introduction

This book is about the nurturing, training and strengthening of bones. What a bizarre idea! Why should we care about our bones, unless we have the misfortune to break one? The truth is that bones – like teeth, skin and hair – slowly decay with age, although we are unaware of the fact because they are hidden beneath layers of skin, fat and muscle. The process of decay is extremely slow. The results – fractures and skeletal deformities – may not declare themselves until the seventh decade of life, or later.

Why, then, do we now hear such a lot about osteoporosis? After all, there have been old people around for centuries. There are two answers to this question. The first and most important is that we are living longer. The extension of human life is one of the great achievements of twentieth-century medicine. In the United States, for example, a white male baby born in 1900 had a life expectancy of 48.2 years and a white female baby a life expectancy of 51.1 years. A person who expects to die at the age of 50 does not need to worry about osteoporosis or any other age-related degenerative disorder. In 1984 the life expectancies of white babies in America were 71.8 years for boys and 78.8 years for girls, an increase of more than 50 percent in less than a century. Similar statistics are found in other developed countries. Average lifespan has increased because infant mortality has been drastically reduced and because fewer of us now succumb to infectious diseases. All of this has been achieved through a combination of preventive medicine – massive immunization programs, better personal and environmental hygiene – and the invention of more efficacious drugs.

The impact of these changes becomes even more evident when one looks at the numbers of people attaining old age. In 1900, out of 1,000 babies born in the United States, only 470 were expected to live to the age of 60 and only 160 were expected to reach the grand age of 80. In 1980 these figures were 890 and 410 respectively. This trend has caused a large increase in the relative size of the elderly population, not just in the United States but throughout the developed world. Again taking the United States as an example, at the end of this century there will be nearly four times as many old people, as a percentage of the total population as there were at the beginning of it. In 1900 the over-65s represented 4 percent of the American population, in 1980 they made up 11.3 percent, and in 2040, if the present trend continues, one in five Americans will be aged 65 or over.

It is hardly surprising, therefore, that disorders which were comparatively rare when most people died at around the age of 50 are now more prevalent and more worrying to the general public and to the medical profession. Some of these disorders, such as atherosclerosis (the narrowing and hardening of blood vessels), are fatal and can cause premature death. Others, although seldom fatal, cause pain, disability, dependence, and a marked decrease in the quality of life for millions of old and elderly people. Osteoporosis belongs to this group.

Like many of the internal processes of aging, osteoporosis starts quite early in life, in the fourth decade in fact, but there are no external symptoms until much later, not until the seventh or even eighth decade perhaps. These internal processes tick away unseen, so we do not worry about them, unlike changes in skin, hair and fat distribution, for which we have developed a whole arsenal of creams, cosmetics and diets. The external manifestations of osteoporosis – shortening stature, back pain, a gradual hunching of the spine, and fractures – appear when it may be too late to do anything about it.

Like other age-related disorders, osteoporosis is part of a slow, natural decline in the functional capacity of the body, but it is also a symptom of poor health habits. Its onset and progress can be accelerated by an unbalanced diet, lack of exercise, smoking, and various other factors. Like other disorders of later life, osteoporosis is also progressive and universal. The older you are the more likely you are to be affected, and men as well as women can be affected, although usually at a later age. Lastly, and this too is a feature of age-related disorders, the rate at which osteoporosis progresses can be remarkably different in different individuals. Some people progress rapidly to severe disability, while others remain symptom-free, or rather free of obvious external symptoms, throughout their lives.

These characteristics have important implications when it comes to thinking of ways to combat osteoporosis. The obvious conclusion is that a preventive approach is likely to be more successful than prophylactic, after-the-fact intervention. The stable door must be bolted before the horse has a chance to escape. If a process which is at least partly natural cannot be prevented, it can at least be delayed for as long as possible.

Epidemiologists gloomily refer to this approach as the "compression of morbidity."

Which brings us to the second group of reasons for the current high profile of osteoporosis. In the last decade several accurate, safe and comparatively cheap methods of estimating bone mass, and therefore bone loss, have been developed. Early detection of osteoporosis is now possible, and the effects of various treatments can also be assessed with a very small margin of error. This does not mean that everyone approaching the age of 50 should start asking for these tests. But if you belong to one or more of the risk groups listed on page 120, you should consider doing so. If your bone mass is found to be below normal for your age and build, a choice of treatments is open to you. Increasing your physical activity and making sure your diet contains sufficient calcium are usually considered to be *preventive* measures, but there are indications that both strategies can arrest or at least slow down the osteoporotic process once it has begun. Exercise and calcium are maximally effective in adolescence and early adulthood, building up the reserves of bone on which we draw in later life. The other option is medication, in the form of estrogen and other drugs. These are usually prescribed when bone loss is already evident.

The main message of this book is that physical activity can prevent and slow down the osteoporotic process. Bone is a living tissue and its growth is stimulated by mechanical stress. The exercises presented in the central section of this book, which "load" certain bones in ways which stimulate their growth, are based on the results of recent research with women *already* suffering from osteoporosis. The effects of exercise on younger women are therefore likely to be even more positive. The details of this research are given on page 136, but the good news is that repeated, regular loading of specific bones can and does increase bone mass by a significant amount. In the study just referred to, a control group of women who did not do bone-loading exercises continued to lose bone mass.

In the second half of the book the reader will find a more detailed description of the rationale behind bone-loading exercise and also answers to some of the most frequently asked questions about osteoporosis.

In osteoporosis, as in many other ailments, all of us have two broad choices: we can take a measure of responsibility for our own health by becoming reasonably informed and by taking simple preventive measures, or we can sit tight and call the doctor when the disease is already upon us and perhaps too far advanced to treat.

exercise *program*

Why exercise? Far from depleting our energies, exercise adds energy to body tissues and to the mind and spirit. It boosts intellectual performance, self-esteem, self-confidence, emotional resilience, resistance to stress, resistance to illness. . . . It reminds the body of the range of activity it is capable of, from total relaxation to strenuous effort. Too many of us exist in a state of moderate tension most of the time, somewhere in the middle of our potential range, and we maintain that state of tension for so long that it becomes the norm and eventually traps us into illness, or into mental and emotional cul-de-sacs.

Physical exercise is, after laughter, the best medicine. Taken regularly, in moderate doses, and within physiological limits, it has no negative side-effects. As far as osteoporosis is concerned, exercise is both preventive and prophylactic. But not just any exercise. To be effective against osteoporosis, exercise must bend, compress, twist and stretch specific bones in slightly unusual ways. New bone is laid down in response to such stresses.

Bone-loading can be used to build bone reserves and therefore postpone or prevent serious bone loss, or it can be used to help reverse or delay the rate of bone loss once osteoporosis has begun. But remember, **if you have been diagnosed as having a moderate or severe degree of osteoporosis, exercise must be very controlled and gentle to start with** (the tests which measure loss of bone substance are described on pages 128–132). **If you suspect you have osteoporosis or that you are particularly at risk, consult your doctor** (risk factors are listed on pages 119–123).

The bone-loading exercise program
The exercises in this book are mainly for women aged 35 or over, and especially for those who are physically inactive or only active on a sporadic basis. They contain aerobic and anaerobic elements − aerobic exercises get the heart and lungs working and build up stamina, and anaerobic exercises are usually done with weights or against some other form of resistance and they increase muscle power − and also exercises which improve flexibility, coordination and balance. But the main focus is on exercises which improve bone status.

Five groups of exercises are presented: warm-ups, stretch and flexibility exercises, bone-loading exercises, back and tummy toners, and cool-downs, and this is the order in which they should be done. Please, please, please never do bone-loading exercises without having stretched and warmed up first. Warm muscles and connective tissue are less vulnerable to injury.

The bone-loading exercises (pages 48–99) start from five basic positions: standing, sitting on a chair, kneeling on all fours, sitting on the floor, and lying on the floor. We recommend that you do two or three exercises in each position to start with and that you vary the exercises you do at each session. The more variety the better. Start with standing exercises, then chair-sitting exercises, then descend to floor level. This gradual progression could be important if you suffer from postural hypotension (feeling faint when you get up from a sitting or lying position).

Many of the movements involved in the bone-loading exercises will feel unfamiliar. This is the whole point of bone-loading. Living bones respond to the mechanical demands made on them, and the more unusual those demands are the more positively they respond.

After the bone-loading exercises come exercises for the abdomen. Weak abdominal muscles and a protruding belly go with poor posture, and poor posture spells backache whether you are skinny, normal or overweight. By working on your tummy muscles, you can de-stress your back muscles.

Every bone-loading session should end with a cool-down routine. This allows your heart to slow to its normal rate and returns you, composed and alert, to whatever you are doing.

Some dos and don'ts To make your bone-loading sessions safe, comfortable and effective, here is a summary of what you should and should not do:

- Start slowly, go gently, and if you get very out of breath or something hurts, STOP IMMEDIATELY. Always work within your level of fitness (see page 20).
- Always warm up at the start of a session.
- After a few warm-ups, work through the stretching and flexibility exercises; then you will be ready to start bone-loading.
- Do two or three bone-loading exercises from each section – graduating from a standing position to sitting on a chair, kneeling on all fours, sitting on the floor, and finally lying on the floor.
- Try the first few bone-loaders in each section to begin with – they're the easiest – and choose different bone-loaders at each session.
- Don't worry if you cannot manage the required number of repetitions to start with – that will come later.

- Start gently and always work rhythmically, but remember that you are supposed to be LOADING your bones, so a certain amount of vigor is in order.
- Do bone-loading exercises for the spine, femurs and forearms at each session – don't concentrate on single bones.
- Don't forget to breathe! Where there are no instructions about inhaling and exhaling, breathe as smoothly and naturally as you can. Don't be tempted to hold your breath when the exercise is difficult – your muscles need the oxygen. At moments of peak effort, try talking or counting out loud – that will stop you holding your breath.
- Always do a few back and tummy toners after the bone-loaders.
- Allow yourself a minute or two of complete relaxation at the end of the session.

How long should sessions be and how often? The times given below are only a rough guide since a lot depends on your level of fitness (see next paragraph).

Exercise times in minutes

	Beginners	Intermediate	Advanced
Warm-ups	1	3	4
Stretch/flex	1	3	4
Bone-loaders	5	10	15
Back/tummy	2	3	5
Cool-downs	1	1	2
Total	10	20	30

To be effective, bone-loading exercises should be done at least three times a week or every other day.

How fit are you? The best way of finding out how much exercise you can safely do is to have a medical check-up – blood pressure, electrocardiogram (ECG) at rest and during exercise, blood tests, and so on. **If you are over 40 or have not been physically active for some time, or only intermittently, you should consult your GP before embarking on this or any other exercise program. Even if you feel perfectly fit and well, play safe and ask for a check-up.**

When you exercise, your heart has to work harder, so before you start it is important to establish what your maximum safe heart rate is. The radial artery pulsing in your wrist will tell you how fast your heart is beating. At rest, 70–80 beats a minute is average for non-athletes over the age of 40, but at peak effort the heart may have to work more than twice as hard.

Maximum safe heart rate during exercise is usually calculated as being 190 minus the age of the person concerned. So if you are 50 and your ECG is normal, your maximum heart rate will be 190 minus 50, which is 140. You should never exceed this rate. If your ECG is not normal, ask your doctor what your maximal heart rate should be.

If you experience chest pain or breathlessness during any of the exercises, stop immediately. You may have exceeded your maximum safe heart rate. Try to get into the habit of taking your pulse at the start of an exercise session and at the end of it to make sure that your heart has returned to its normal resting rate.

To take your pulse, place your fingertips on the inner side of your wrist on the thumb side and feel the throbbing of the radial artery. Look at a clock or watch with a second hand and count the number of beats for 15 seconds and multiply by 4. That will give you the number of beats per minute.

Improving general fitness Although the exercises in this book will do a lot to improve the health of your bones, and your flexibility, coordination and balance, they should be complemented by other activities which improve aerobic function. Here are some of the everyday things you could do to keep your heart healthy:

● Use your legs. Park your car further away from the office/shops or, if you use a bus, walk one stop before boarding and get off one stop before your destination.
● Use the stairs rather than the elevator or the escalator – you'll probably get there quicker!
● If you spend a lot of time sitting down, kick your legs from time to time, pull your tummy in, squeeze your buttocks together, get up and stretch, take a few deep breaths ... anything to get your blood moving!

If you swim, jog, dance, cycle or play a ball or raquet sport, so much the better. If you are not very fit, start with three 10-minute sessions a week and gradually work up to three 30-minute sessions. A little and often is a better policy than a lot infrequently.

Clothing and other equipment Wear a loose top and jogging pants, preferably of cotton, and sneakers. Bare feet are not recommended, except for foot and ankle flexibility exercises, because they tend to slide on carpet.

Some of the exercises in this book require a stout stick – a broomstick will do. Others use a belt or piece of rope. A few use small weights – if you cannot buy mini dumb-bells or wrist or ankle weights, improvize your own. Cans of beans make very adequate lightweight dumb-bells, and wrist and ankle weights can be made out of fabric filled with sand. Floor work is also more comfortable if you use an exercise mat, thin mattress or folded blanket.

Some of the traction exercises can be done, most enjoyably, with a partner, but a few require some form of exercise ladder or a few transverse bars placed at strategic heights in a doorway – two possible solutions are suggested on page 152. Whether you set up your apparatus against a wall or in a doorway, it should be strong enough to take all or most of your weight and the wall or doorway must be very solid. It does not take much imagination to realize that hanging onto doors and unsecured items of furniture could lead to nasty accidents. Rather than take that risk, choose exercises which do not involve the ladder – there are plenty to choose from.

A creative solution to the ladder problem might be to form a bone-loading group and work out in a local gym! Exercising in a group often does more for morale and perseverance than exercising solo.

WARM-UPS

Why warm up before exercise? The main reason is that warmed-up muscles are flexible muscles and less vulnerable to injury than cold muscles. The aim of warming-up is not to build muscular strength or stamina but to get the heart pumping faster and more forcefully so that more blood reaches every part of the body, especially the skeletal muscles. Blood contains oxygen, and working muscles need many times more oxygen than resting muscles; if they don't get it, cramp can set in.

How much warming up should you do? Well, enough to cause you to perspire and be a little short of breath, but not so much that you have to pant or gasp for breath . . . enough to push up your resting heart rate by 20–30 beats per minute. If your resting pulse rate is 75 beats per minute, warming up should take you to 100–105 beats per minute.

Try to inhale through your nose and exhale through your mouth. In fact it is best to inhale twice, in two short breaths, and exhale in one long blow. Practice doing that before you start.

Warm-ups are more enjoyable with music in the background, especially music with a beat which makes you want to move or dance to it. The tempo should be one you can comfortably exercise to.

As with all other forms of exercise, start slowly and become familiar with the movements before you try to speed up or do lots of repetitions. One minute of warming up is probably enough for beginners, but this is something you will have to judge for yourself. If you are not perspiring or only moderately out of breath at the end of one minute, keep going for a little longer. Advanced bone-loaders should warm up for at least three minutes.

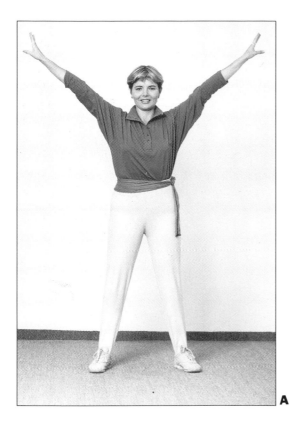

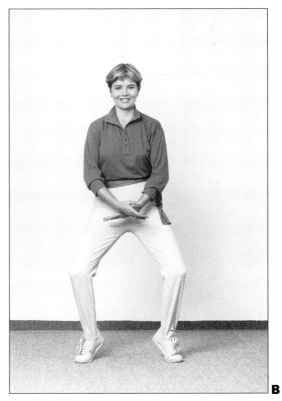

WARM-UP 1

A Stand erect, feet shoulder-width apart and pointing outward, arms raised above head, palms down. Inhale.

B Swing arms down so that hands cross in front of stomach, bend knees and raise heels. Exhale.
Repeat A and B, inhaling and exhaling, for at least 1 minute. Work up a comfortable rhythm.

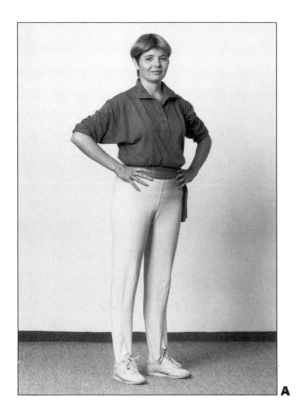

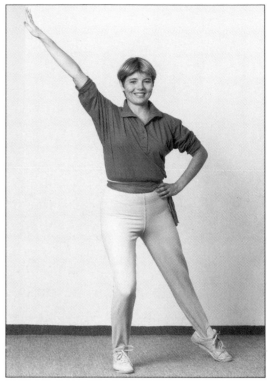

A

B

WARM-UP 2

A Stand erect, feet comfortably apart, hands on hips.

B Extend right arm and left leg in opposite directions, slightly bending right knee. Inhale. Return to start position A and exhale.

C Repeat with left arm and right leg. Inhale. Return to start position A and exhale.

D Extend right arm up and forward and left leg back, bending right knee. Inhale. Return to start position A and exhale.

E Repeat with left arm and right leg. Inhale. Return to start position A and exhale.

Repeat vigorously and rhythmically, in time with your breathing, for at least 1 minute.

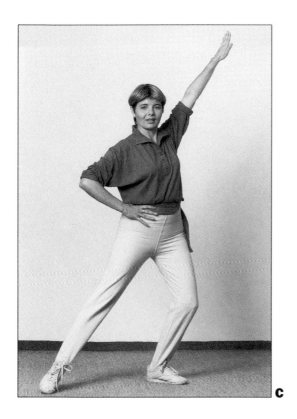

C

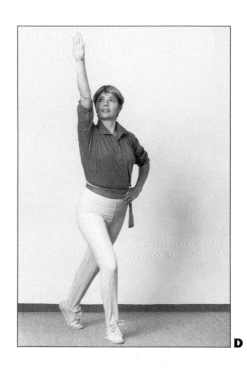

D

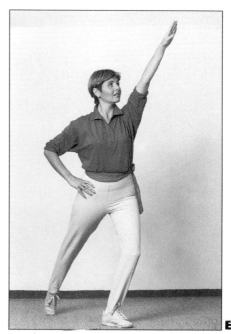

E

WARM-UP 3

For this exercise you have to imagine there
is a solid wall on either side of you, just
beyond arm's reach.

A Stand erect, feet a little more than
shoulder-width apart, hands on shoulders,
elbows out to sides. Inhale.

B Without moving your feet, twist to the
right, with front knee bent and back knee
straight, and push on the right hand wall
with your left hand. Exhale. Return to start
position A and inhale.

C Now twist to the left and push on the
other wall with your right hand. Exhale.
Return to start position A and inhale.
Repeat right and left wall pushes to the
count of four, in time with your breathing,
and continue for at least 1 minute.

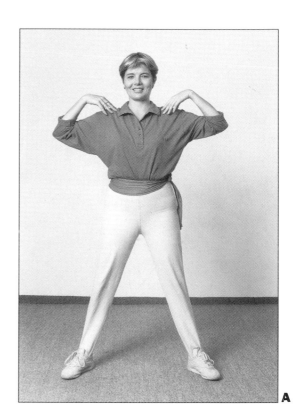

A

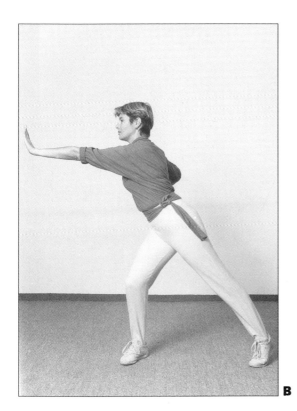

B

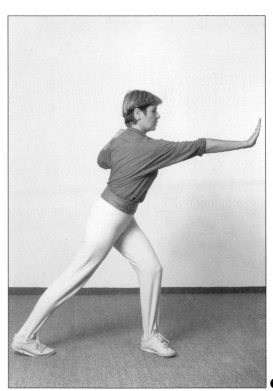

C

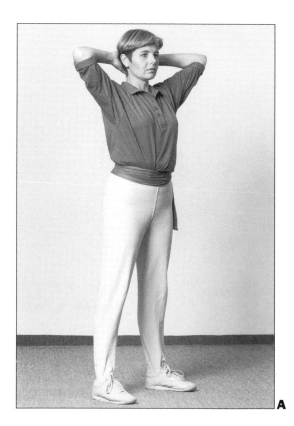

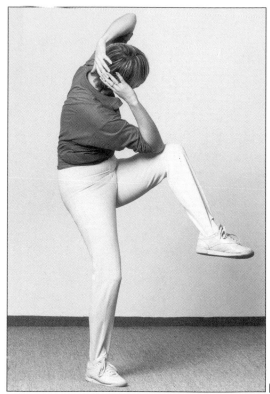

WARM-UP 4

A Stand erect, feet shoulder-width apart, hands clasped behind neck, elbows open wide. Inhale.

B Raise left knee as high as you can and twist torso so that right elbow meets raised knee – try to keep your elbows out! Exhale. The aim here is to *twist* rather than bend the back. If knee and elbow don't meet, don't worry, and don't be tempted to bend your back – your twistability will increase with practice!

Return to start position A and inhale.

C Raise right knee and try to touch it with left elbow. Exhale. Return to start position A and inhale.

D Bend left knee as if to touch buttocks with heel, and touch heel with opposite hand. Exhale. Return to start position A and inhale.

E Repeat so that left arm touches right heel. Exhale. Return to start position A. Inhale. Repeat the whole sequence, continuing for at least 1 minute.

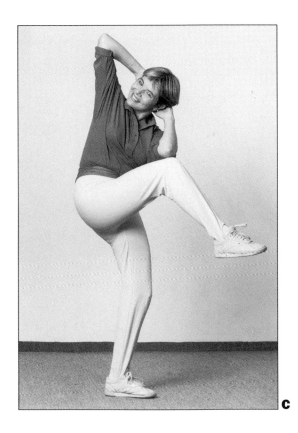

C

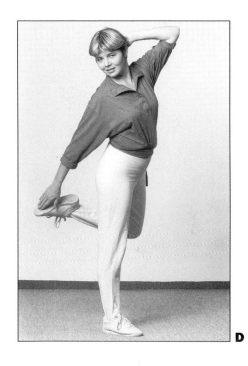

D

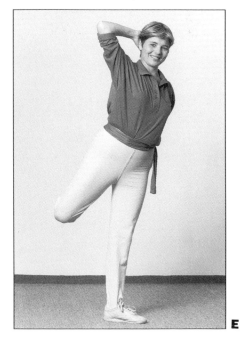

E

WARM-UP 5

This is really jogging/running on the spot.

A Jog gently on spot, arms held loosely, heels touching floor with each step. Jog for 1 minute, breathing as naturally as possible. If this feels comfortable, proceed to B, but if it makes you feel very breathless, stop and check your pulse.

B Run on spot, lifting knees higher. Your elbows should be bent and your hands loosely clenched. Make sure your heels touch the floor with each step. Continue for 1 minute. If this feels comfortable, continue for 2 minutes.

C Decrease speed and effort and revert to gentle jogging for 30 seconds, then walk around the room for 15 seconds. Rest. Kick each leg a few times and breathe deeply before moving on to the stretching/flexibility exercises.

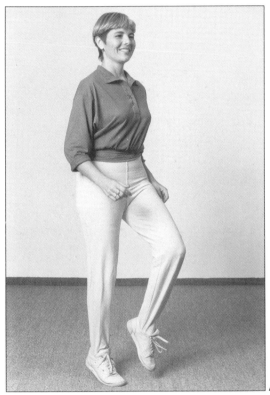

A

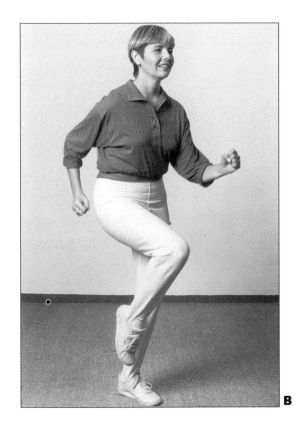

B

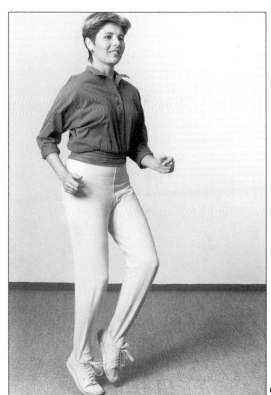

C

STRETCH/FLEX EXERCISES

Muscles work best when their ends are farthest apart, but they can be injured if they are not properly warmed up and stretched first. That is why stretching is an integral part of any pre-exercise routine. Stretching increases the flexibility of muscles and connective tissue and give joints a greater range of movement.

The slow, sustained stretches described in this section lengthen muscles without exceeding their elastic limit. Stretching should never be fast or forced – no pumping or bouncing movements to achieve more of a stretch! If you do that your muscles will automatically tighten in order to protect themselves and their joints against injury.

So always do stretching exercises slowly, concentrating on the muscles and joints you are working on. Visualize one set of muscles lengthening while another set shortens – simply thinking "length" into a muscle has a definite effect. The rest of you should be as relaxed as possible. Breathe naturally – no holding your breath when you reach the limit of a stretch. Keep breathing and you will probably find that you can stretch a little further.

Try to hold each stretch for a few seconds. The benefit of this is that during a stretch the muscles that are being stretched slowly relax, and once the stretch is over the muscles that have been contracted also relax. After a few stretches and holds you will probably feel a very pleasant sensation of warmth. That's good.

In this section there is an emphasis on balance. Standing on one leg, or on your heels or toes, not only strengthens the muscles involved but also improves your ability to shift your body weight quickly – very important when the unexpected happens. Lack of agility, slow reactions and poor coordination lead to many accidents, even in young people.

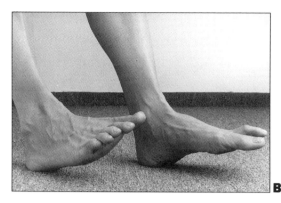

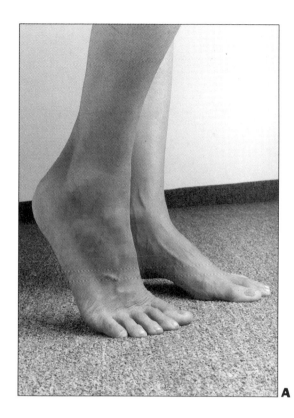

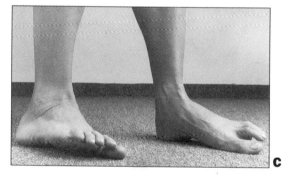

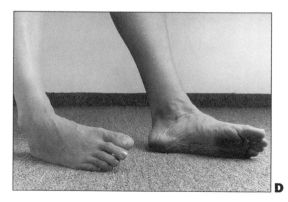

STRETCH/FLEX 1

feet

These exercises are best done with bare feet
– shoes only restrict movement.

A Walk 20–30 steps forward on toes, then
backward.

B Walk forward and backward on heels.

C Walk forward and backward on inside
edge of feet.

D Walk forward and backward on outside
edge of feet.

STRETCH/FLEX 2

ankles

These exercises should be done standing next to a chair or table, but do not hold onto it unless you lose your balance. As soon as you regain your balance, let go.

A Stand on one leg, raise the other and, keeping raised knee as still as possible, point big toe inwards.

B Point big toe outwards.

C Point big toe up.

Now draw imaginary circles with your toe, the wider the better, first clockwise, then anticlockwise. Repeat standing on the other leg.

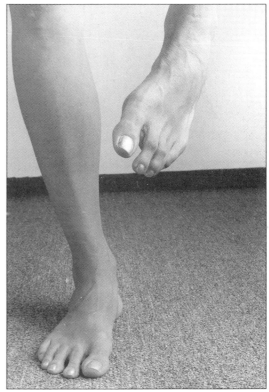

A

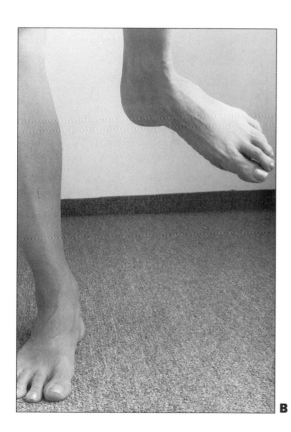

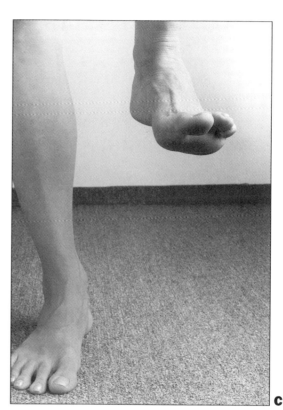

STRETCH/FLEX 3

thighs

Stand next to a chair, right hand on hip, left hand just touching the chair for balance.

A Raise right knee to waist level.

B Swing knee out to side.

C Raise heel towards buttock – imagine foot being pulled up toward ceiling.

Now draw imaginary circles with your knee, the bigger the better, first in one direction, then in the other. Repeat standing on the other leg.

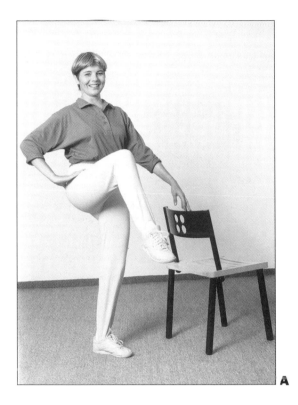

A

STRETCH/FLEX 4

hands

A Clench both hands into fists, and hold for a few seconds.

B Stretch fingers as wide apart as possible and hold for a few seconds.

Remember to keep breathing! Repeat clenching and stretching 10 times.

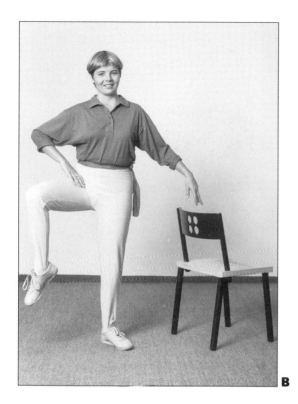

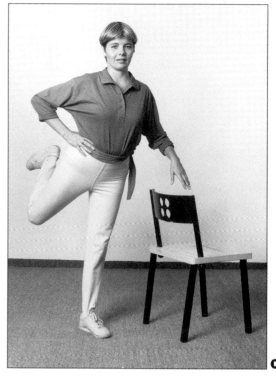

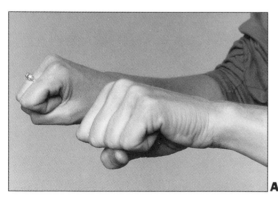

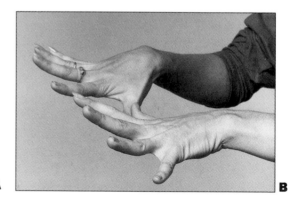

STRETCH/FLEX 5

wrists

A Keeping elbows bent but still, point fingers down as strongly as possible and hold for a few seconds.

B Point fingers in as strongly as possible and hold briefly.

C Point fingers up as strongly as possible and hold briefly.

Now, still keeping elbows and forearms as still as possible, draw imaginary circles with your fingers, first in one direction, then in the other. Repeat 8 times in each direction. If you notice a marked difference, concentrate on the wrist that seems stiffest.

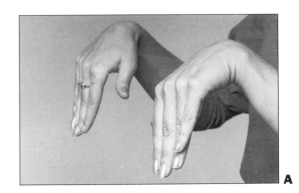

A

STRETCH/FLEX 6

shoulders

A Stand erect, arms overhead, left hand holding right elbow.

B Gently reach down back with right hand while left hand pulls right elbow back.

Return to start position A.

Repeat 10 times with each hand.

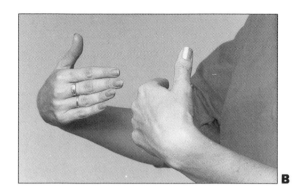

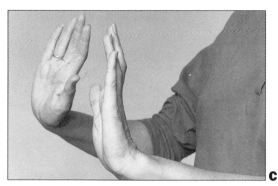

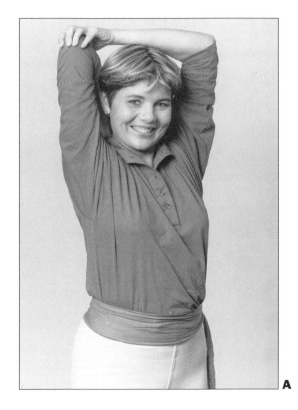

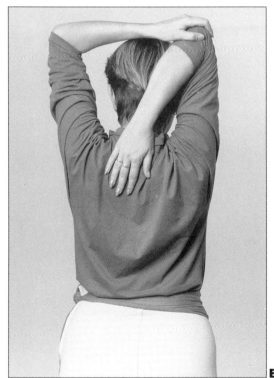

STRETCH/FLEX 7

shoulders

A Sit on a chair, back straight, legs slightly apart, hands clasped behind the back of the chair.

B Straighten arms behind you and raise them as far as is comfortable, allowing neck and torso to tip forward slightly. Hold for a few seconds. Relax arms and return to start position A.

Repeat 10 times.

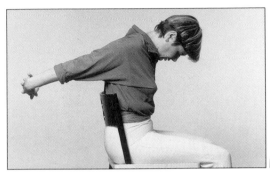

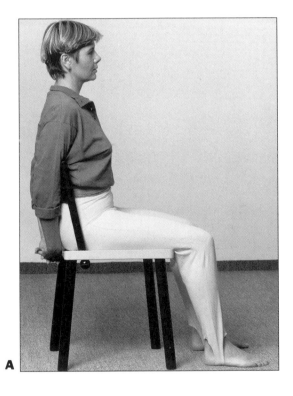

STRETCH/FLEX 8

neck

This exercise can be done sitting or standing. All movements should be slow and unforced – the weight of the head is quite sufficient to stretch the muscles at the sides and back of the neck. Hold each position long enough to release tension. Do not roll your head backward!

A Start position – head up, chin level.

B Sidebend neck as if to touch left shoulder with left ear.

C Let head roll forward.

D Roll head towards right shoulder as if to touch it with right ear. Return to start position A.

Repeat 5 times left to right, and 5 times right to left.

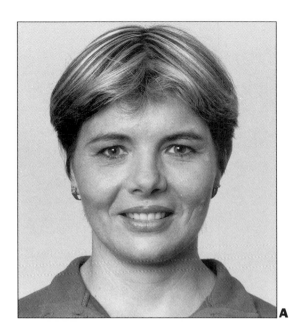

A

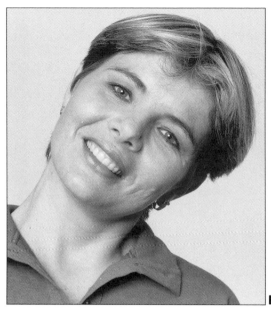

B

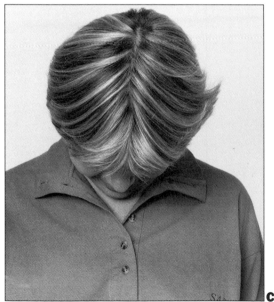

C

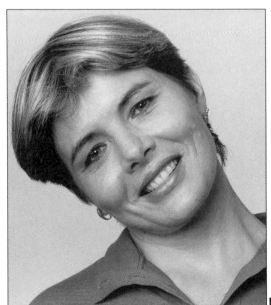

D

STRETCH/FLEX 9

neck

This exercise can also be done sitting or standing.

A Start position – head up, chin level.

B Without moving shoulders, slowly turn head to look over right shoulder.

C Slowly turn head to look over left shoulder.

Repeat several times until your neck feels loose and relaxed.

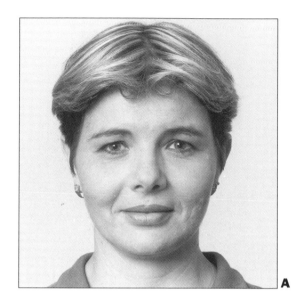

A

STRETCH/FLEX 10

waist

A Stand erect, feet parallel and shoulder-width apart, hands on hips.

B Rotate pelvis back, pull in stomach, and squeeze buttocks together. Return to start position A and relax.

Repeat 10 times.

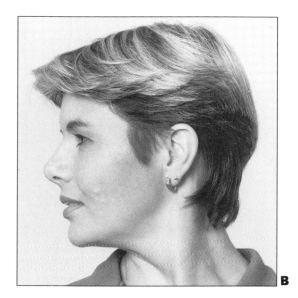

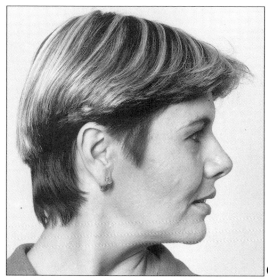

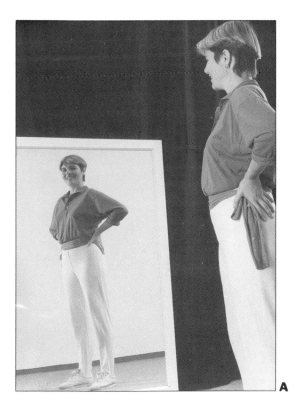

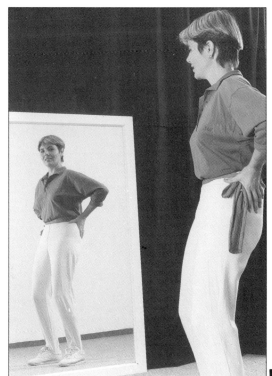

STRETCH/FLEX 11

waist

A Stand erect, feet parallel and shoulder-width apart, arms straight out in front, hands clasped.

B Without moving feet, turn shoulders, arms and neck to the right as if they were all in one piece. This will ensure a good twist at the waist. Hold for a few seconds, breathing naturally.

C Bending knees slightly, turn even further to right. Hold briefly, breathing naturally. Return to start position A and repeat on other side.

Compare twisting to the right with twisting to the left – one side will probably feel easier than the other. Work harder with the restricted side.

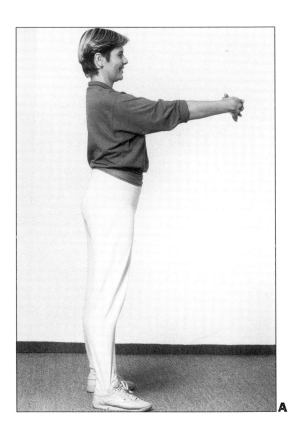

A

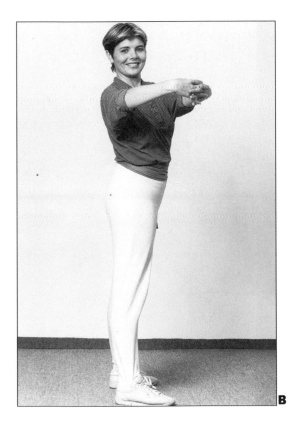

B

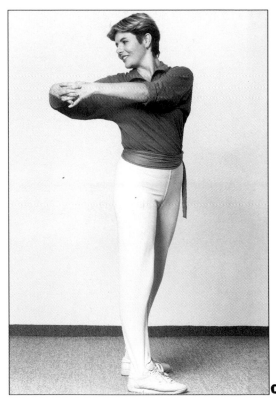

C

STRETCH/FLEX 12

general

A Stand back to back with partner, feet shoulder-width apart, arms stretched out to sides, holding hands. Keep holding hands!

B Keeping arms as straight as possible and without moving feet, raise one arm over head, turn torso in other direction and let other arm swing down between you.

C Bend knees slightly, allow back heel to leave floor and continue circling arms until you and your partner are chest to chest. Hold this position for a few seconds and smile at your partner!

D Circle your arms back the way you came.

E Continue circling until you have returned to start position A.

Now go through the same sequence on the other side. Repeat gently 10 times on each side. Mutual coordination is called for, but it's a lot of fun!

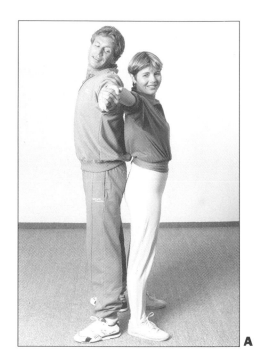

A

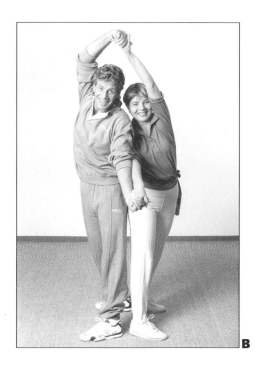

B

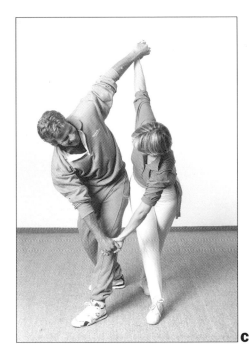

C

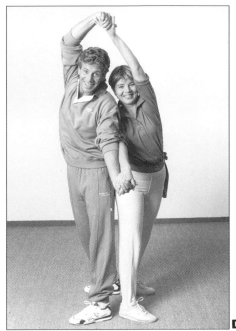

D

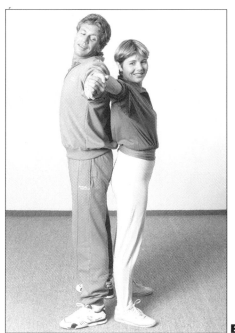

E

BONE-LOADING EXERCISES

Here we come to the core of the exercise approach to osteoporosis. The exercises which follow are designed to load those bones most susceptible to collapse and fracture when they become osteoporotic. Those bones are mainly, but not exclusively, the spinal vertebrae, the femur (thigh bone) and the radius (the bone on the thumb side of the forearm). These bones are highlighted in the drawing on page 117.

As the Jerusalem study proved – if you turn to page 136 you will see how the study was conducted and the results it achieved – only loads which are diverse, slightly unusual and swiftly and repetitively applied are effective in building and restoring bone density. In other words, osteoporosis can only be prevented or combatted by exercises which bend, stretch, twist and compress bones in ways which are not normal in everyday life. This is why walking and jogging, beneficial as they are to the cardiovascular system, are not very effective against osteoporosis – they simply compress the bones of the legs and spine in the same old way. You will not find any compression loading exercises for the spine or femur in this book. What the bones really need to encourage the deposition of new bone are new mechanical messages. The exercises which follow provide lots of new messages.

The exercises are numbered 1–43 and are divided into five sections: standing, sitting on a chair, kneeling on all fours, sitting on the floor, and lying on the floor. All of these positions provide opportunities for using specific muscles, and therefore bones, in new ways.

In each section the early exercises are less strenuous than the later ones. So, to start with, try the first two or three exercises in each section.

The number of repetitions is important – the Jerusalem study showed that only repeated loading during the same session is effective – but increase the number of repetitions slowly.

Variety is also important. Don't concentrate on just one bone – work on the spine, radius and femur at every session, and if you find one side of your body more restricted than the other, give that side some extra work.

Think in terms of 5 minutes of bone-loading per session at first, and gradually work up to 15–20 minutes. If you become short of breath, slow down a bit and try to breathe more deeply and rhythmically. Check your pulse to make sure you are not exceeding your maximum heart rate.

BONE-LOADERS standing

While you are doing these exercises, think about your posture – neck long, chin neither up nor down, collarbones lifted, stomach pulled in, pelvis tilted back, coccyx low, knees very slightly bent, weight somewhere between heels and toes . . .

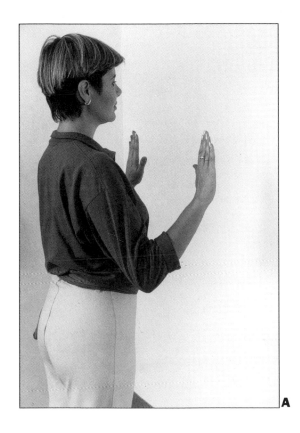

A

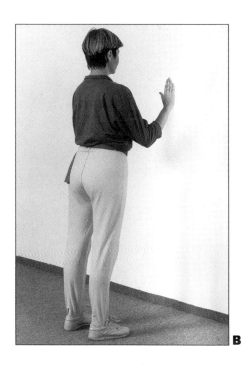

B

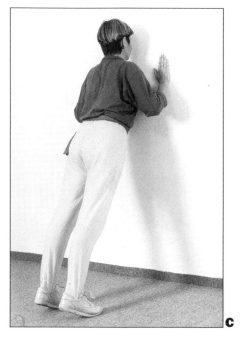

C

BONE-LOADER 1

compression and bending of forearms

A Stand facing wall, toes about 20 inches/50 cms away from it. Position palms at shoulder height half way between chest and wall.

B Keeping legs and body in a straight line, fall towards wall, controlling fall with hands. Push yourself back to start position A.

C If that felt comfortable, repeat exercise, but this time stand a little farther away from the wall.

Repeat 10 times.

BONE-LOADER 2

traction of forearms

A Stand close to ladder, facing it, hands holding rung just below shoulder level.
B Keeping legs and body in a straight line, fall away from ladder, preventing fall by hanging on with your hands. Pull yourself back to start position A.
Repeat 10 times.

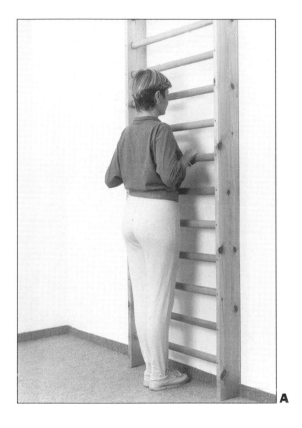

A

BONE-LOADER 3

traction and bending of spine, traction of forearms

A Face your partner, your feet parallel and shoulder-width apart. Your partner, with one foot in front of the other, grasps you by the wrists. As you bend your knees, curl your back, rotate your pelvis back and pull your stomach in, your partner pulls firmly on your arms. Feel the stretch in your arms and spine. Straighten up.

B Stand sideways on to your partner, feet together, arms raised above head. Bend sideways towards your partner so that he/she can grasp your wrists. Push your hips away from your partner and feel the stretch. Straighten up.
Repeat both exercises 5 times on each side.

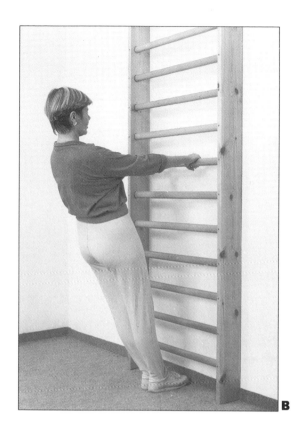

B

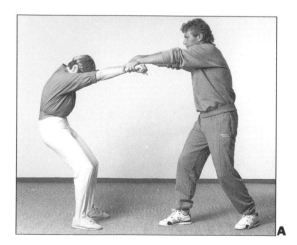

A

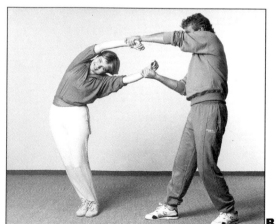

B

51

BONE-LOADER 4

traction of arms and spine

A Stand on lowest rung of ladder and reach up to grasp highest rung.

B Take feet off lowest rung and hang from hands. Try to relax legs and spinal muscles. Feel the stretch throughout your body. Breathe as naturally as possible. Return to start position A and step down from ladder. Repeat 5 times.

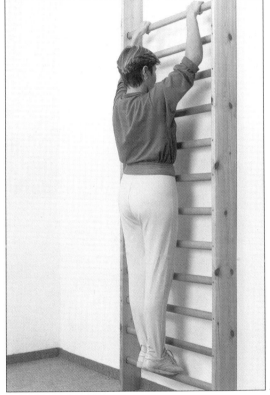

A

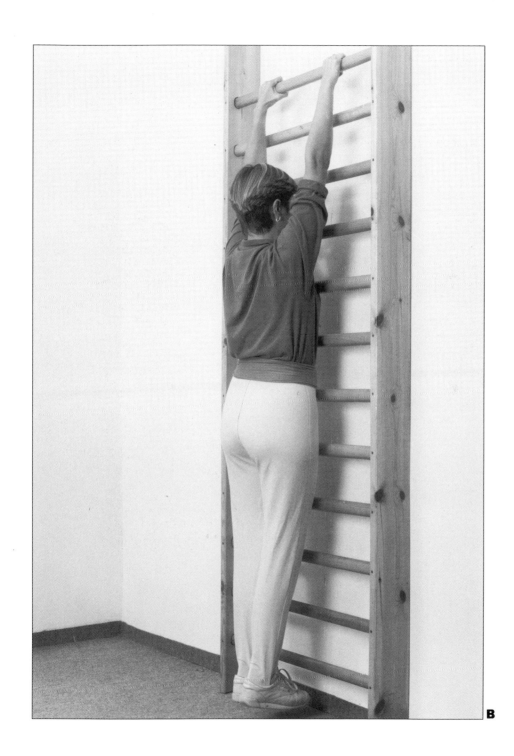

B

BONE-LOADER 5

bending forearms in various planes

A Fold belt in two and hold it in front of you at shoulder level, hands fairly close together. Pull on belt as if to stretch it, and hold for 5 seconds. Relax.

B Raise belt above head and pull hard for 5 seconds. Relax.

C Repeat with belt behind back.

D Repeat with belt behind neck.

Keep breathing! Repeat 5 times in each position.

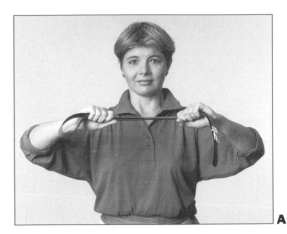

A

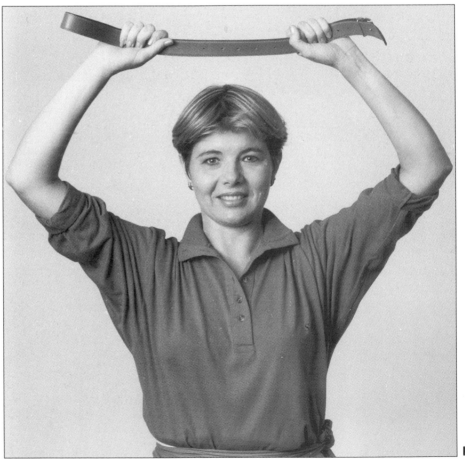

B

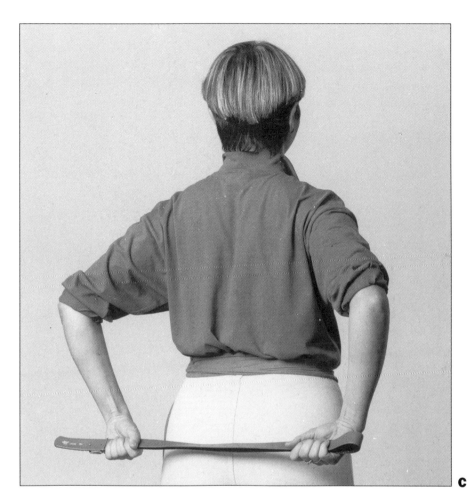

C

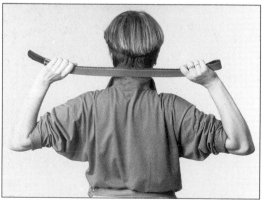

D

BONE-LOADER 6

traction of spine and forearms, bending of femurs

A Stand facing ladder, feet shoulder-width apart, toes pointing outward. Hold the rung at head level.

B Bend knees, keeping kneecaps over toes. Rotate pelvis back as if there were a heavy weight suspended from the bottom of your spine. Feel the stretch in your arms and spine. Hold for 5 seconds. Return to start position A.

C Move your hands down a rung and repeat. Then down another rung and repeat, until your buttocks touch the floor. After a bit of practice your buttocks will reach the floor even when your hands are on a higher rung. That's how much you've stretched!

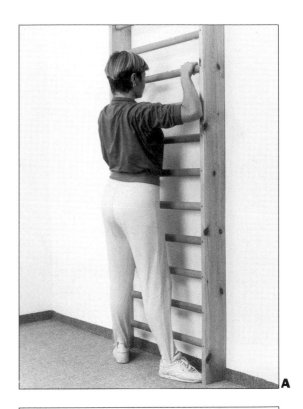

A

BONE-LOADER 7

torsion of forearms

A Face your partner. Hold each other's wrists and twist forearms in opposite directions against partner's resistance. Hold the twist for 5 seconds, then relax. Repeat twist in opposite direction.

B Still facing your partner, grasp right wrists only, and twist in opposite directions. Hold twist for 5 seconds, then relax. Repeat twist in opposite direction. Change hands and repeat.

Repeat both exercises 10 times.

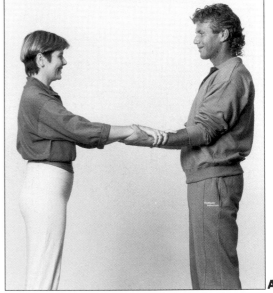

A

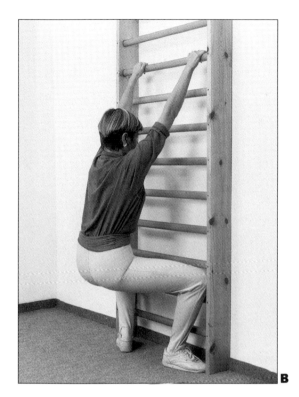

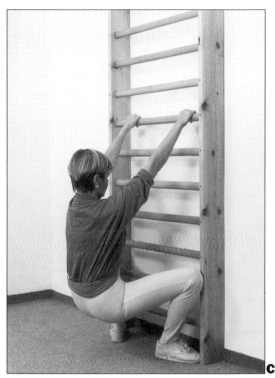

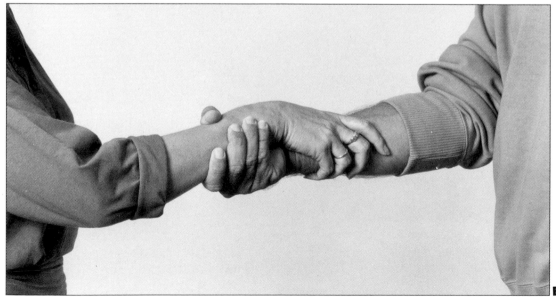

BONE-LOADER 8

bending forearms

A Face your partner. Both of you grip a stout stick at both ends, palm above at one end and palm below at the other (see photograph).

B Now imagine yourself "wringing" the stick by rotating the ends in opposite directions. Your partner resists you by wringing the stick the opposite way. Repeat, trying to wring the stick in the opposite direction.

Now change the position of your hands and repeat.

Repeat both exercises 10 times.

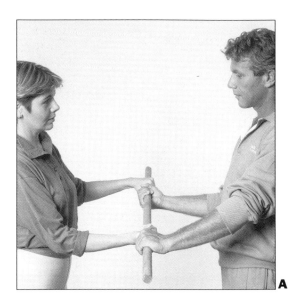

A

BONE-LOADER 9

sidebending spine

A Strand erect, feet shoulder-width apart.

B Slide right hand down right thigh and bend sideways – imagine you are bending between two flat panes of glass. Bend the left elbow so that it points to the ceiling. Breathe naturally. Return gently to start position A, then sidebend to left.

Repeat 15 times on each side, alternating sides.

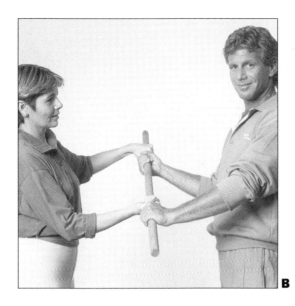

B

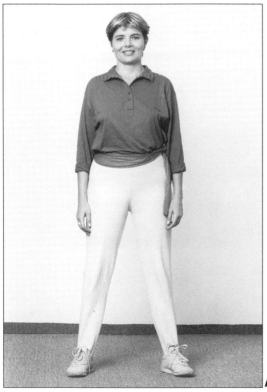

A

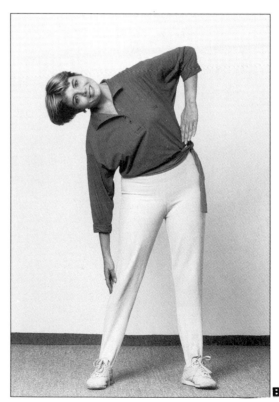

B

BONE-LOADER 10

sidebending spine

A Stand sideways on to ladder, holding rung just below shoulder level with your left hand and rung above head with right hand. Move hips away from ladder so that right arm straightens. Hold for 4 seconds, then relax.

B Move right hand to a lower rung. As before, move hips away from ladder, keeping legs straight. Hold for 4 seconds, then relax. Repeat both exercises 10 times, then change to other side and repeat 10 times.

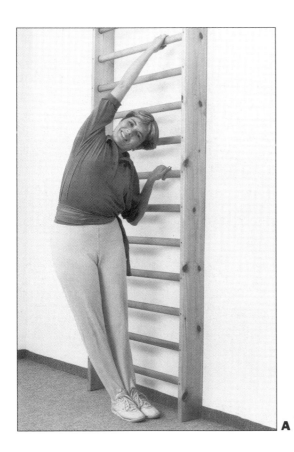

A

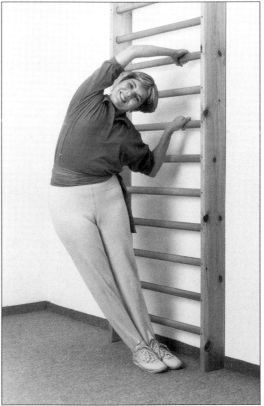

B

BONE-LOADER 11

bending and torsion of femurs

A Stand with feet parallel and shoulder-width apart, knees slightly bent.

B Without moving toes, raise heels and turn them inward.

C Lower heels to floor so that they meet, like Charlie Chaplin's.

D Raise heels again, and this time turn them out as far as you can.

E Lower heels to floor. Return to start position A.

Repeat whole sequence 15 times, as vigorously and smoothly as you can.

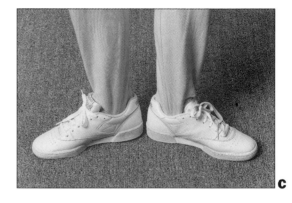

C

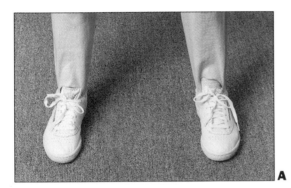

A

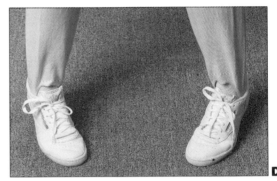

D

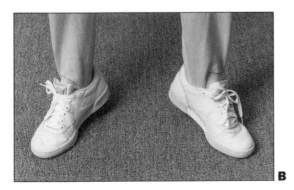

B

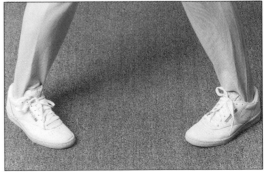

E

BONE-LOADER 12

bending and torsion of femurs

A Stand with feet parallel and shoulder-width apart, knees slightly bent.

B Without moving heels, raise toes and turn them inward.

C With heels still in the same place, stand with your toes touching.

D Raise toes, pivot on heels and turn toes outward as far as you can.

E Lower toes and stand with feet pointing in opposite directions.

Repeat whole sequence 15 times.

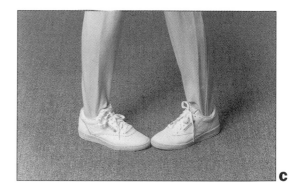
C

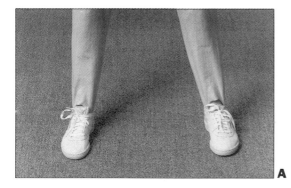
A

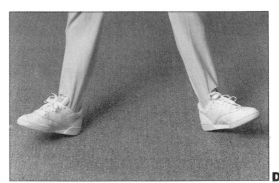
D

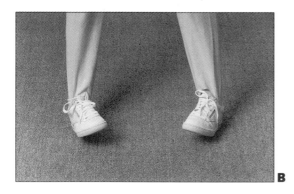
B

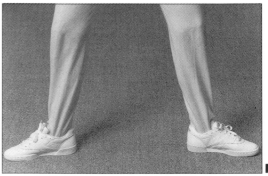
E

BONE-LOADER 13

bending forearms in various planes

In this exercise, by changing the position of your hands and elbows different bending stresses are applied to the forearms.

A Stand at arms' length from wall. Place palms on wall.

B Keeping back and legs in a straight line, and elbows by sides, push yourself toward the wall, controlling the movement with your hands, then push yourself back up to start position A. Repeat rhythmically 10 times. Now change position of palms and elbows (fingers pointing towards each other, elbows out). Keeping back and legs in a straight line, fall towards wall, then vigorously push yourself away from it. Repeat 10 times.

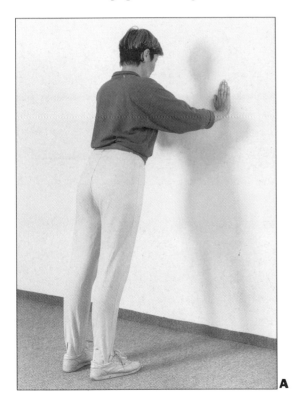

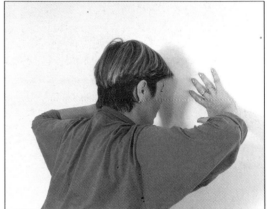

BONE-LOADER 14

bending femurs and spine

A Stand sideways on to ladder so that you can just reach it with of your left hand. Grasp a rung at shoulder level with your left hand and put your left foot on a rung at mid-calf level, keeping your foot parallel with rung.

B Keeping both legs straight, swing your right hand over your head and reach for a rung above your head. Hold for 4 seconds, then relax. Change sides and repeat. Repeat 10 times on each side.

C If this is comfortable, place your foot on a higher rung and repeat 10 times on both sides.

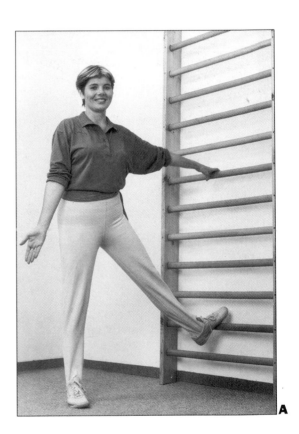

A

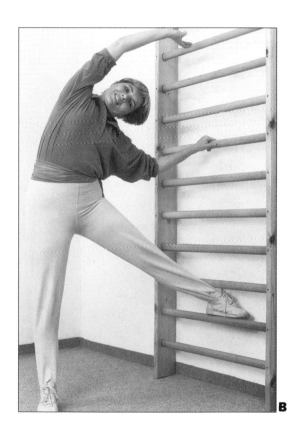

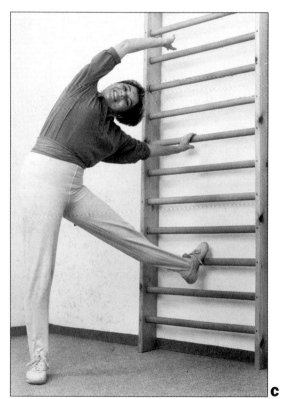

BONE-LOADER 15

torsion of spine and traction of forearms

A Stand back to back with partner, about 2 feet/60 cms away from each other. Both of you now turn to the same side, toward each other, without moving your feet.

B Hold hands and try to turn your shoulders away from each other. This should create a strong pull on your arms. Return to start position A.

C Both of you now turn to the other side, hold hands and try to turn away from each other. Return to start position A.

D Now turn toward each other, grasp each other's far wrist, and try to turn back to start position A. Repeat on other side.
Repeat each of the above 5 times.

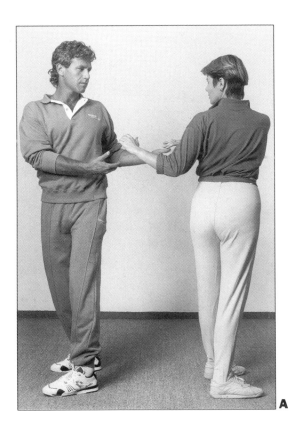

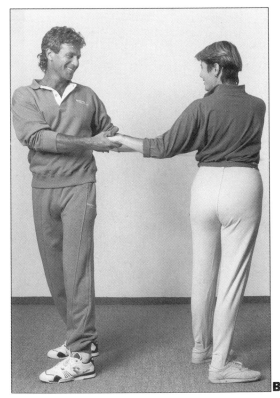

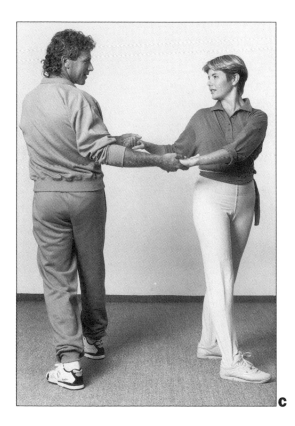

C

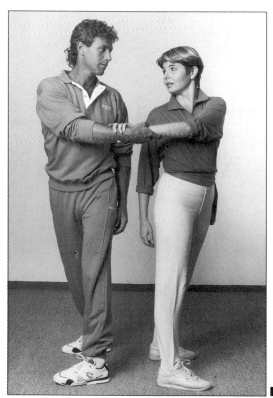

D

BONE-LOADERS
sitting on a chair

What could be easier than exercising on a chair? But make sure the chair is really strong and solid, with a straight, supportive back and no arms. If you suffer from low back pain, you should always sit in a chair which supports your lower back.

The partnered exercises on pages 72, 73 and 74 are the most fun.

BONE-LOADER 16

bending and torsion of spine

A Sit in chair, arms hanging loose, back well supported. Inhale.

B Bend sideways as if to touch floor with right hand. Exhale. Slowly return to upright position, and inhale. Now bend to the other side, reaching towards the floor with your left hand. Exhale. Repeat 10 times on each side, alternating sides.

C Now reach down towards the floor with both hands, but do not let your buttocks come off the seat. Exhale. Return to upright position and inhale. Now reach down on the other side of the chair. Exhale. Repeat 10 times on each side, alternating sides.

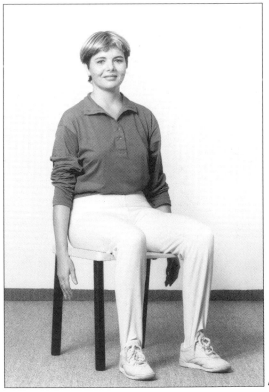

A

BONE-LOADER 17

torsion of spine

A Sit on edge of chair. Without moving buttocks, turn and grasp back of chair, then try to turn away while your hands resist the movement. Hold for a few seconds. Twist around a little further, then try to turn back again. Hold for a few seconds. Repeat on the other side.

Repeat 5 times each side.

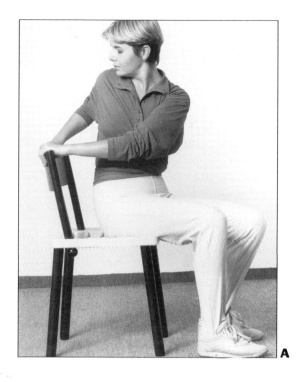
A

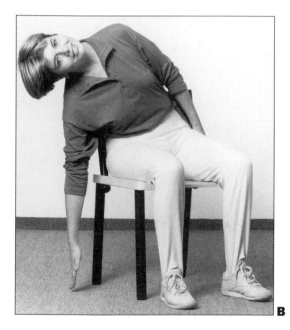
B

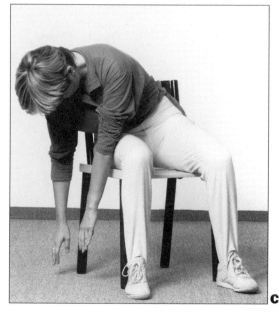
C

BONE-LOADER 18

bending spine

A Sit astride chair, facing and holding onto chair back.

B Rotate pelvis back – imagine a piece of string pulling your waist back – and straighten arms. Hold for a few seconds, then rotate pelvis forward and return to start position A.

Repeat several times.

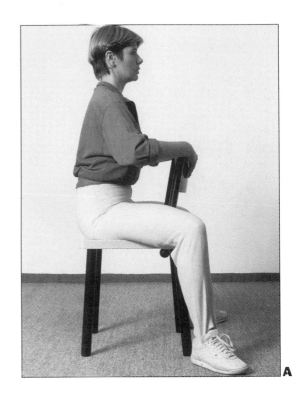

A

BONE-LOADER 19

tension, compression and torsion of forearms

A Place palms together at chest level, with elbows raised. Inhale. Push palms together hard for 5 seconds, and exhale as you do so. Release and inhale. Repeat 12 times.

B Link fingers at chest level, elbows out to sides. Exhale. Pull hard in opposite directions for 5 seconds, inhaling as you do so. Release and exhale. Change the way your fingers are linked, and repeat. Repeat 12 times in all.

C Raise hands and elbows to shoulder level and hold yourself by the wrists. Twist forearms in opposite directions. Hold for 5 seconds, exhaling as you do so. Change wrist grasp and repeat.

Repeat 12 times.

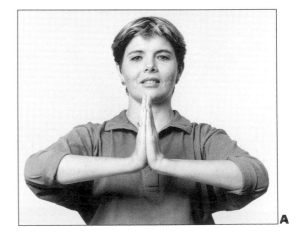

A

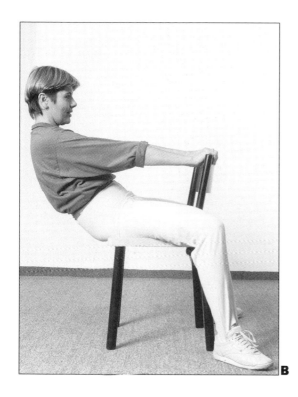

B

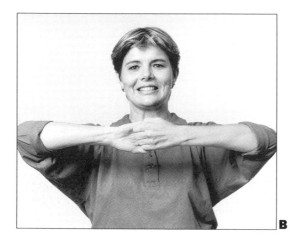

B

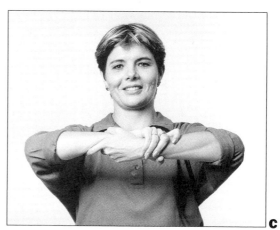

C

BONE-LOADER 20

bending femurs

A Sit facing partner so that your knees are outside his/hers. Grasp seat of chair and push your knees together against your partner's resistance.

B This time your knees are inside your partner's. Push them apart against his/her resistance.

Repeat both exercises 10 times. Talk to each other so that you are not tempted to hold your breath!

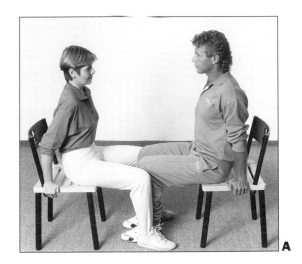

A

BONE-LOADER 21

bending forearms

A Sit facing partner. Put your left hand on your right knee and, bending forward slightly, put your right elbow in your left palm. Your partner does the same. Now grasp your partner's right hand and attempt to arm wrestle it towards your left knee! Breathe! Change arms.

B If you practice hard enough, you might even beat your partner. Even if you don't, it's a lot of fun! Repeat before meals!

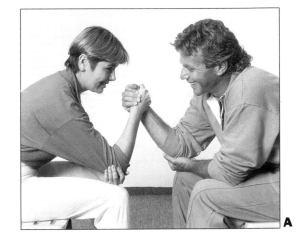

A

BONE-LOADER 22

torsion of forearms

A Hold a stout stick at chest level, with palm-up grip. Inhale. Now try to break the stick by bending both ends toward the ceiling, exhaling as you do so. Relax and inhale.

B Now hold the stick with palm-down grip and try to break it by bending both ends toward the floor.

Repeat both exercises 8 times.

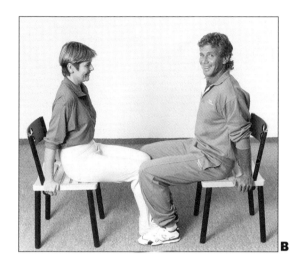

B

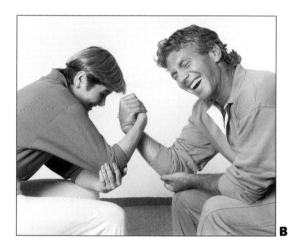

B

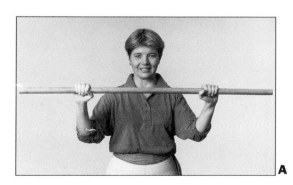

A

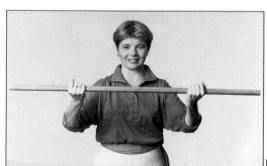

B

BONE-LOADER 23

torsion of spine

A Sit sideways on chair, grasping long stick behind shoulders. Partner stands behind.

B Without moving pelvis, twist shoulders as far to the right as you can.

C Partner grasps stick and tries to turn you further to the right.

D You now try to turn back against your partner's resistance.

Repeat 6 times on each side.

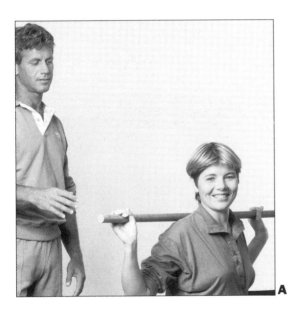

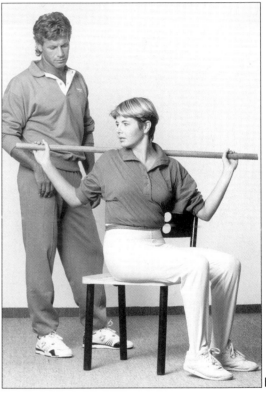

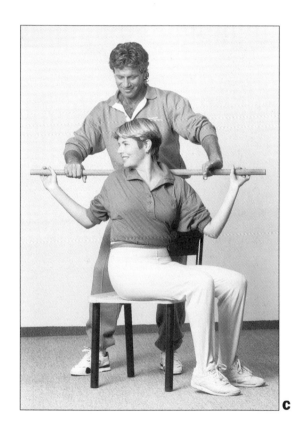

C

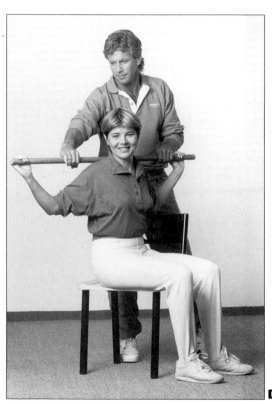

D

BONE-LOADERS on all fours

The starting position for all of the exercises in this section is kneeling on all fours, with arms and thighs vertical to the floor, like the legs of a table. Pull your tummy in and DO NOT ALLOW YOUR BACK TO SAG TOWARD THE FLOOR. Keep your head and neck in line with your back, and LOOK AT THE FLOOR, not at the clock, or this book, or your fellow bone-loaders.... Hyperextension of the neck, or arching the neck back, is a movement that should be avoided.

If you find kneeling painful, put a cushion under your knees. If you have arthritis in your fingers, support yourself on your fists rather than your palms if it feels more comfortable. Don't sit back on your heels between exercises; simply roll onto your side and sit up with legs bent for a few moments.

BONE-LOADER 24

compression of forearms, bending femurs

A Kneel on all fours, palms or fists directly beneath shoulders. Straighten right leg behind you.
B Raise right leg, so that neck, back and leg are in a straight line. KEEP YOUR BACK STRAIGHT AND LOOK AT THE FLOOR. Lower leg almost to floor, then raise it again. Repeat 20 times, then switch to other leg and repeat 20 times.

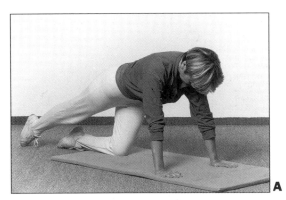
A

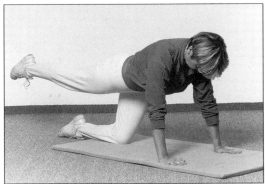
B

BONE-LOADER 25

compression and bending of forearms and femurs

A Kneel on all fours, palms directly beneath shoulders. Place a weight in front of both hands – if you don't have proper weights, use two cans of beans.

B Pick up weight in front of right hand and place it as far ahead of you as you can. Allow your pelvis to move forward slightly, but DO NOT ALLOW YOUR LOWER BACK TO SINK TOWARD THE FLOOR. Pick up the weight and return it to its original position. Repeat with left hand.

Repeat 15 times with each hand, alternating hands. Then try picking up both weights at the same time. Again, do not allow your lower back to sink toward the floor.

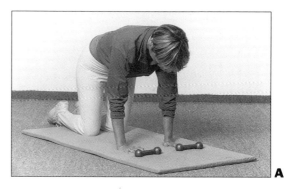
A

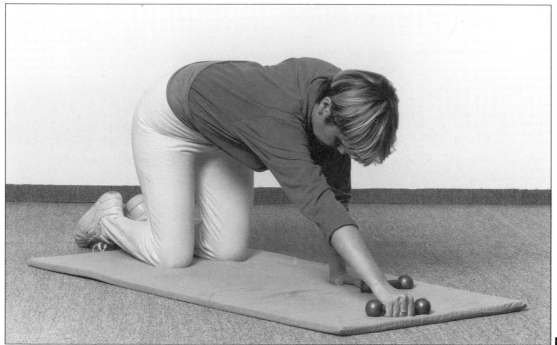
B

BONE-LOADER 26

bending forearms in various planes

A Kneel on all fours, knees and feet slightly apart, hands under shoulders.

B Walk your hands forward, taking small steps, as far as you can reach. Allow your pelvis to move forward slightly but DO NOT HOLLOW YOUR LOWER BACK. Your knees and feet should not move. Walk back to start position A. Repeat 10 times.

C Walk your hands out to the sides, allowing your pelvis to move forward slightly so that your arms and hands bear part of your body weight. Walk back to start position A. Repeat 10 times.

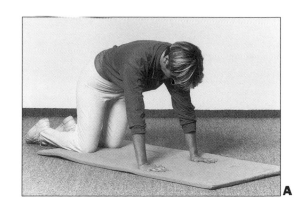

A

BONE-LOADER 27

bending femurs in various planes

A Kneeling on all fours, hands directly under shoulders, extend and slightly raise right leg so that it makes a straight line with your back and neck. Don't rest leg on floor.

B Raise right leg a little further until it is parallel with the floor. DO NOT ALLOW YOUR LOWER BACK TO SINK TOWARD THE FLOOR.

C Bend raised leg at knee and bring knee round to side, keeping knee parallel with floor. Hold for a few seconds. Take knee round to back, straighten leg, and lower to floor.

Repeat 12 times with each leg.

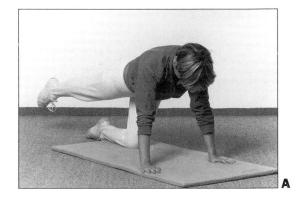

A

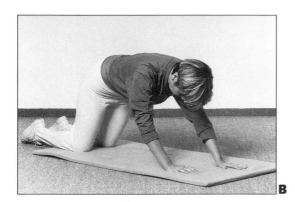

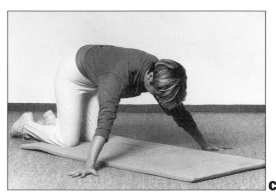

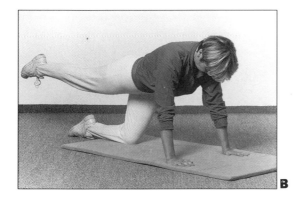

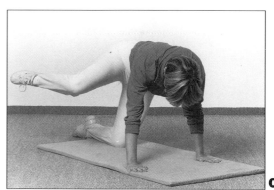

BONE-LOADER 28

traction and bending of femurs

A Kneel on all fours, hands directly under shoulders. Hold weight in crook of right knee.

B Lift right knee so that thigh is parallel to the floor and toe points to ceiling.

C Bring right knee down and forward, rounding your back, tucking your chin under and pulling your stomach in.

Repeat 5 times with each knee.

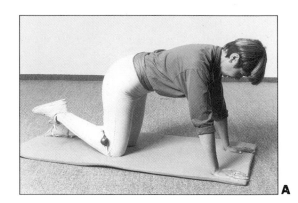

A

BONE-LOADER 29

compression and bending of forearms

In this exercise the head is lowered below waist level. If you suffer from postural hypotension, this exercise should be omitted.

A Kneel on all fours, hands directly under shoulders. Inhale.

B Bend arms at elbows and slowly lower your torso as if to touch the floor with your nose. Reach as far in front of you as you can. Allow your pelvis to move forward but DO NOT ALLOW YOUR LOWER BACK TO HOLLOW. Push yourself back to start position A.

Repeat as many times as you can. This is a woman's push-up. When you feel you have enough strength in your arms, try a man's push up – lie flat on your stomach, toes on floor, palms on floor level with shoulders, and . . . push up, keeping back and legs in a straight line. Takes some doing!

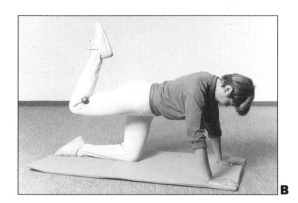

B

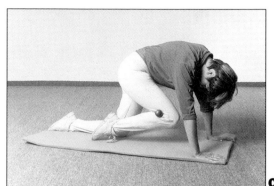

C

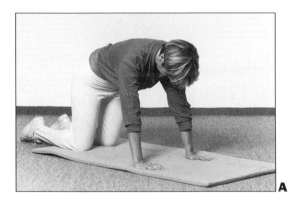

A

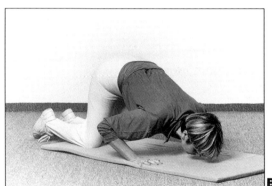

B

BONE-LOADERS sitting on the floor

Since sitting on the floor without a back support is difficult and tiring, all the exercises in this section use a support of some kind – a wall, a partner, your own arms. Most of these exercises apply unique loads and strengthen muscles which are not active in other postures.

BONE-LOADER 30

bending spine

A Sit with back against wall, knees half bent, knees and feet together, arms extended to sides, holding weights (cans of beans will do if you don't have weights). Inhale.

B Bend trunk sideways to right, rolling weight away from you with a straight arm. Reach as far as possible, keeping your buttocks firmly on the floor. Hold for a few seconds. Exhale. Gently straighten to start position A and inhale.

C Sidebend to left, rolling the weight as far away from you as you can. Exhale. Return to start position A and inhale.

Repeat 15 times on each side, alternating sides.

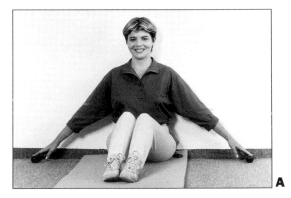

A

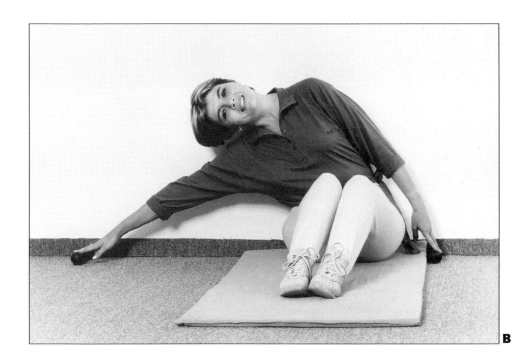

B

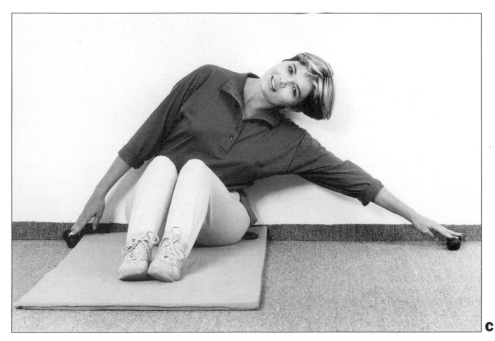

C

BONE-LOADER 31

traction of spine and forearms

A Sit on floor with your back supported against the side of your partner's leg. Your partner grasps your right arm firmly by the wrist and pulls toward the ceiling, maintaining the pull for 5 seconds while you inhale. When your partner stops pulling, lower your arm and exhale.

B Repeat with other arm.

C Raise both arms so that your partner can pull on both. Hold the pull for 5 seconds and inhale. Relax and exhale.

Doesn't that make you feel a little taller? Repeat a few more times.

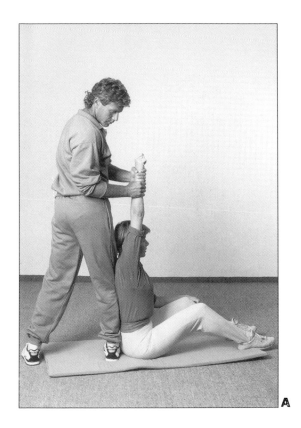

A

BONE-LOADER 32

traction of forearms and bending spine

A Sit facing ladder, with toes on lowest rung and hands grasping rung at shoulder level. Inhale.

B Rotate your pelvis back – imagine that your waist is being pulled back – and lower your chin onto your chest. Allow your arms and spine to stretch. Exhale. Return to start position A and relax.

Repeat 8 times.

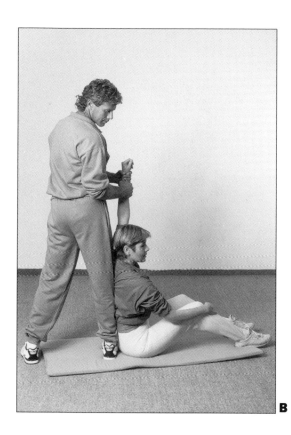

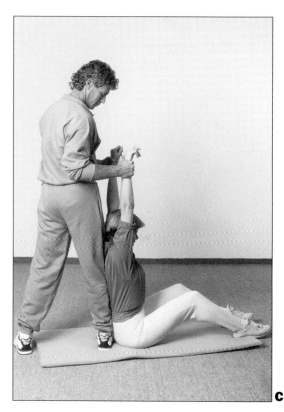

B

C

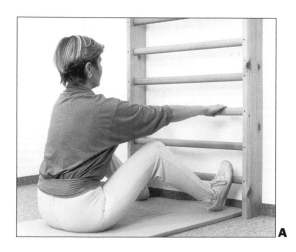

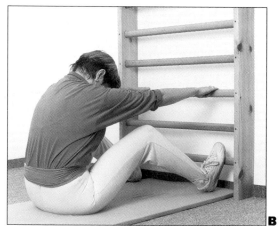

A

B

BONE-LOADER 33

bending femurs

A Sit against wall, knees apart, soles of feet together and as close to groin as possible, elbows on knees and hands loosely grasping ankles. If you cannot put the soles of your feet together, simply cross your ankles.
B Gently push your knees towards the floor until you feel a stretch in the groin. Do not force it. Hold for 5 seconds, then return to start position A.
Repeat 10 times.

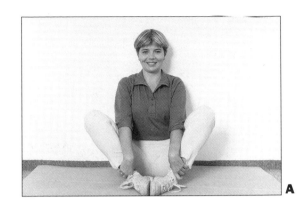
A

BONE-LOADER 34

compression of forearms and bending of femurs

A This may be difficult if you have never tried it before. Sit on floor, place palms of hands on floor on either side of buttocks. Plant soles of feet on floor, shoulder-width apart. Now try to lift your buttocks off the floor. The aim is to lift your body so that it is more or less parallel with the floor. Keep breathing!
B Extend right leg.
C Now raise right leg to hip level, parallel to the floor. Don't hold your breath! Lower leg slowly to floor and return to start position A. Repeat as many times as you can without returning to sitting position. Then rest and repeat with the other leg. If you feel cramp in the back of your thighs, stop. The number of repetitions to aim for is 10 with each leg. That takes some doing, so work up gradually.

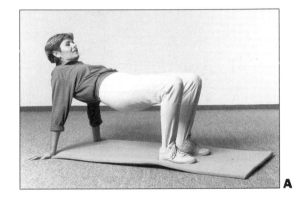
A

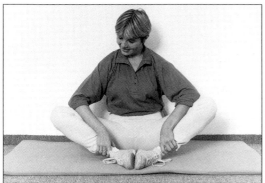

B

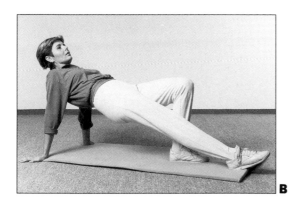

B

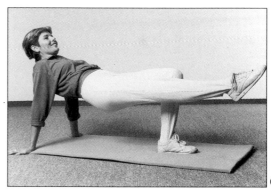

C

BONE-LOADER 35

bending femurs, torsion of spine

A Sit on floor, palms on floor a little way behind buttocks, a weight clamped between your knees. Keeping knees and feet together, lift feet from the floor and lean back onto bent elbows.

B Keeping knees together, roll hips to right.

C Lower knees until right thigh touches floor. Return to start position A and repeat on other side.

Repeat 12 times on each side, alternating sides.

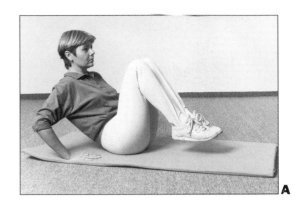

A

BONE-LOADER 36

bending femurs, compression of forearms

A Sit on floor, palms of hands on floor on either side of buttocks. Plant soles of feet on floor, shoulder-width apart. Now lift your buttocks to shoulder level so that your body is more or less parallel to floor. Yes, it's the same start position as in BONE-LOADER 34!

B Using small shuffling steps, walk your feet forward, keeping body and thighs in a straight line. Breathe naturally.

C Keep walking until legs are straight. Hold for a few seconds, then walk back to start position A, keeping buttocks as far away from floor as possible. Sit and rest for a few seconds.

Repeat 8 times.

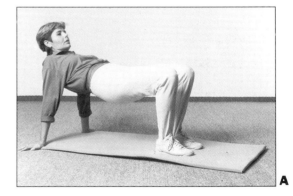

A

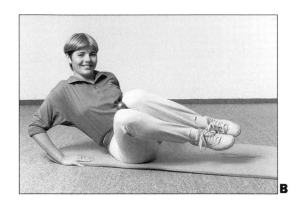

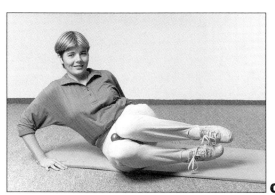

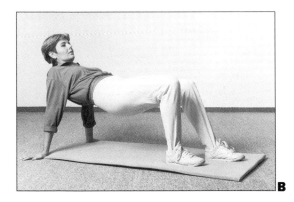

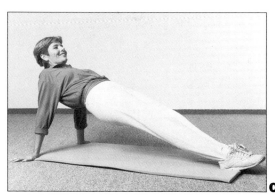

BONE-LOADERS
lying on the floor

In the lying position compression stress is largely taken off the spinal vertebrae and various muscle groups can be exercised in a different relationship to gravity. As the Jerusalem osteoporosis study found, unusual forces exerted on bone have the most potential for increasing bone density.

If you have a marked kyphosis or forward curvature of the upper spine, lying on your back will be uncomfortable unless you put a small pillow or a folded towel under your head. Drop your chin and feel that the back of your neck is long.

BONE-LOADER 37

bending femurs

A Lie on left side, left hand supporting head, right palm on floor near chest, legs straight.
B Lift right leg. Hold for 5 seconds.
C Gently lower right leg – don't let it fall!
D Lift right leg again. Hold for 3 seconds.
E Now lift left leg and attach it to raised right leg. Hold for 3 seconds, then gently lower both legs.
Repeat 10 times on each side.

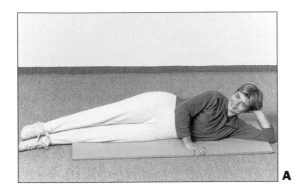

A

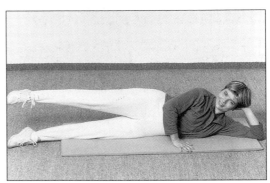

B

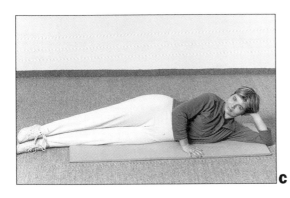

C

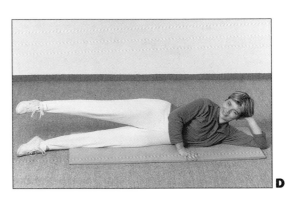

D

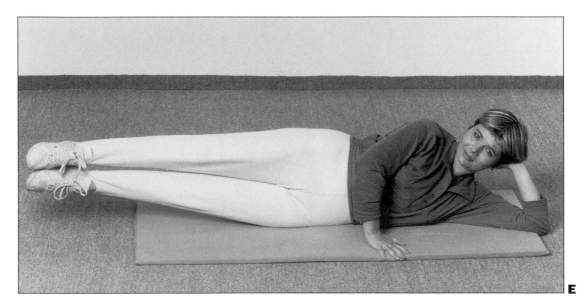

E

BONE-LOADER 38

bending femurs and forearms

A Lie flat on stomach with legs and arms outstretched. Your cheek or forehead should stay in contact with the floor throughout this exercise.

B Lift right leg and left arm. Hold for 5 seconds, breathing naturally. Lower leg and arm – don't let them fall! Repeat 10 times with alternate leg and arm.

C Now lift both legs and both arms. Don't lift your head! Keep breathing. Lower legs and arms slowly. Repeat 10 times.

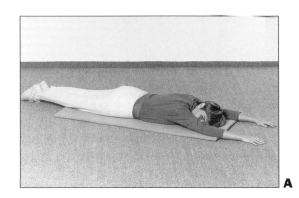

A

BONE-LOADER 39

bending femurs

A Lie on left side, left hand supporting head, right palm flat on floor in front of chest. Left leg should be slightly bent and right knee pulled toward chest, with thigh parallel to floor.

B Raise right knee to ceiling, hold for 5 seconds.

C Scissor right knee backward, keeping knee bent at right angles. Hold for 5 seconds.

D Now rotate right thigh so that toe points to ceiling. Hold for 5 seconds, then return to start position A.

Repeat sequence 10 times on each side.

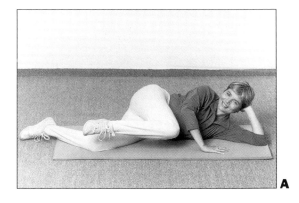

A

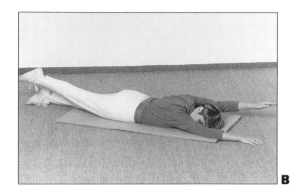

B

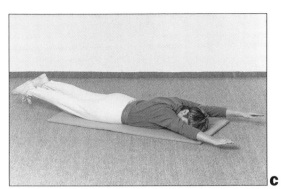

C

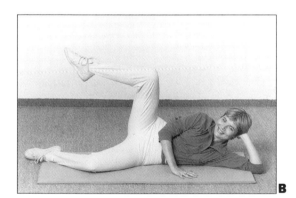

B

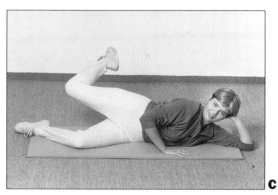

C

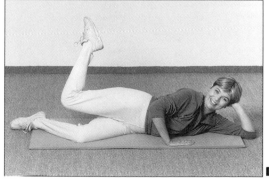

D

BONE-LOADER 40

torsion of spine

A Lie on back, legs straight, arms extended cross-fashion.

B Slowly swing left leg over right until foot touches floor.

C Without moving shoulders, lift left buttock and *drag* left leg toward right arm – bend it a little if you need to. Now *drag* leg back across right leg to start position A. Repeat 8 times with each leg.

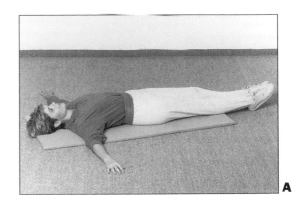

A

BONE-LOADER 41

bending femurs

A Lie on side, left hand supporting head, right palm on floor near chest, left leg slightly bent, right knee pulled toward chest.

B Extend right leg in front of you, with toe a little way off the floor. Hold for 5 seconds.

C Now lift right leg to hip height, hold for 2 seconds, then lower almost to floor. Repeat 15 times.

Repeat 15 times on other side.

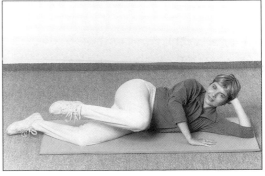

A

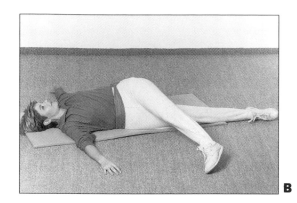

B

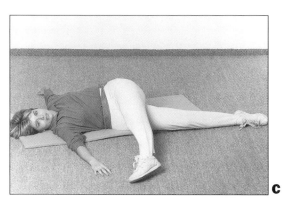

C

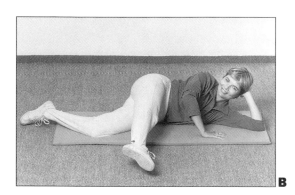

B

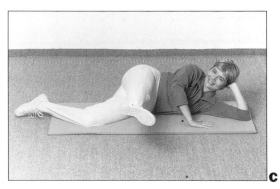

C

95

BONE-LOADER 42

traction of femurs and bending spine

A Partner sits on chair. You lie on your back, holding a stick wrapped in a towel behind your bent knees and grasping the front legs of the chair with both hands.

B Lift your knees towards your partner, who reaches for and holds the stick.

C Your partner gently pulls the stick while you resist, trying to push your buttocks towards the floor. Hold for 4 seconds. Keep breathing!

D Your partner releases his/her hold on stick. You continue to hold buttocks off floor. Now slowly roll your back onto the floor and relax for a few seconds.
Repeat 8 times.

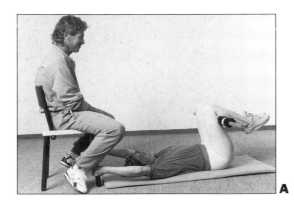

A

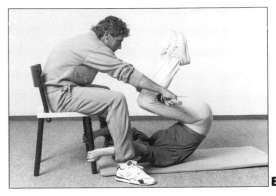

B

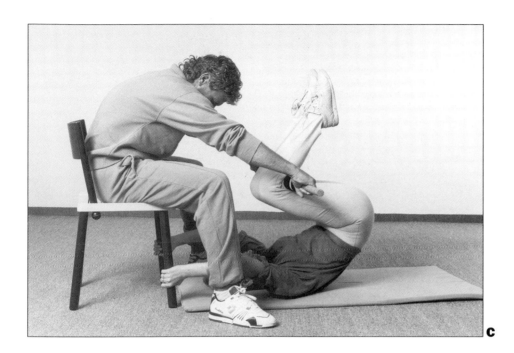

C

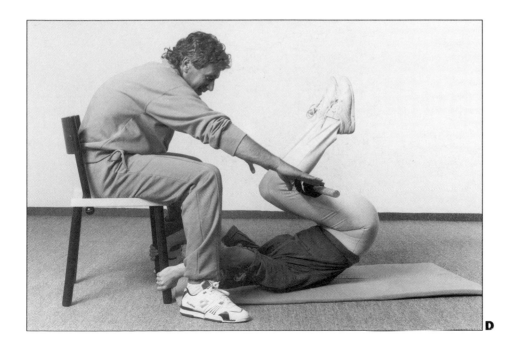

D

BONE-LOADER 43

bending spine and femurs, traction of forearms

A Lie on back in front of ladder, buttocks touching it and legs vertically against it, arms loosely by sides.

B Curl head and shoulders forward, reach toward a low rung and hold for 5 seconds.

C Now reach toward the next rung, and the next, climbing hand over hand . . .

D When you have climbed to the highest rung you can reach, climb back down again to start position A. Repeat 8 times.

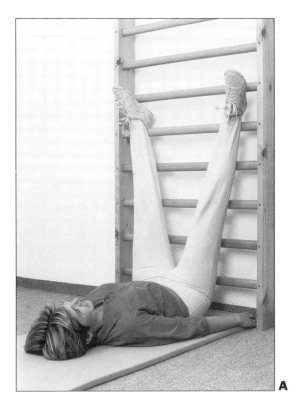

A

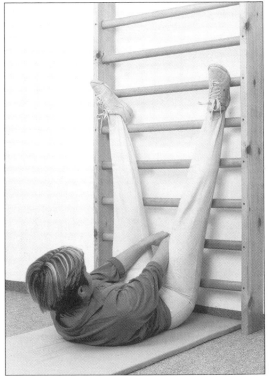

B

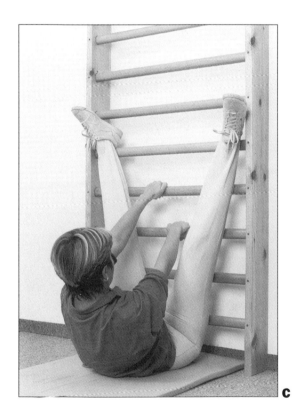

C

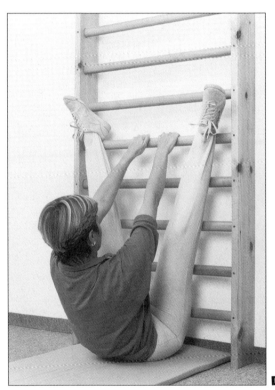

D

BACK AND TUMMY TONERS

Like many other muscle groups in the body, those of the back and abdomen work reciprocally. So by improving the tone of the abdominal muscles, a lot of tension and aching can be taken out of the back muscles. The women who took part in the Jerusalem study which proved the effectiveness of bone-loading exercise in osteoporosis (see page 136) all reported a decrease in back pain as the result of tummy toning exercises.

Although the back muscles, together with powerful muscles in the buttocks and thighs, do most of the work which keeps us upright, the abdominal muscles also contribute to posture. By bracing the abdomen against the back, they keep all the abdominal organs in the right place and also cut down the work of the back muscles.

All of the exercises in this section are done lying or sitting on the floor. The first few are easier than the later ones, but do not despair. Master the easy ones first and slowly work up to the number of repetitions required.

The muscles of the abdomen are attached to the lower ribs and to various parts of the pelvis, and like all muscles they are capable of doing two kinds of work, concentric and eccentric. When working concentrically they progressively contract, bringing the ribs closer to the pelvis; when working eccentrically, they slowly de-contract, allowing the ribs and pelvis to separate in a controlled manner. Eccentric muscle work consumes more energy than concentric, as you will soon find out! The muscles worked on are mentioned at the beginning of each exercise.

BACK/TUMMY 1
straight abdominal muscles

A Sit on floor, left leg straight, right leg bent. Stretch arms out in front and hold belt with both hands at shoulder level.

B Rotate pelvis back and put right foot through hands and over belt, without touching belt. Hold for a few seconds, then return to start position A. Repeat 10 times with each leg.

C Bring belt a little closer to chest, and once again put right foot through hands and over belt without touching it. Hold for a few seconds, then return to start position A. Repeat 10 times with each leg.

D Now, balancing on your buttocks, put both legs through your hands and over the belt without touching it.

E Hold for a few seconds, then reverse the movement. Repeat D and E 10 times, each time drawing your hands a little nearer your chest.

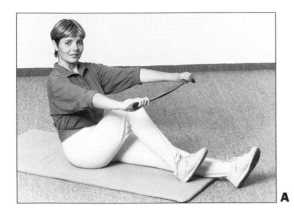

A

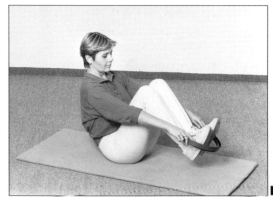

D

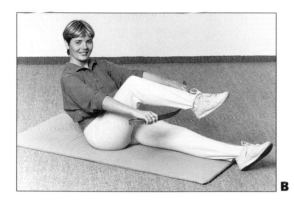

B

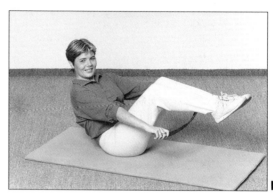

E

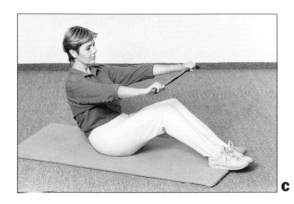

C

BACK/TUMMY 2

straight abdominal muscles

A Lie on back with feet shoulder-width apart and tucked under lowest rung of ladder. Knees should be slightly bent and arms stretched straight forward.

B As you contract your abdominal muscles, curl head and shoulders forward and reach between your knees. Breathe naturally.

C Hold the rung at shoulder level.

D If you can't quite reach the ladder, support yourself on one elbow and reach for ladder with the other hand.

E Let go of ladder and slowly roll back to start position A. Count 1, 2, 3 as you roll back and 4 as you lie down. Rest for a few seconds.

Repeat 12 times.

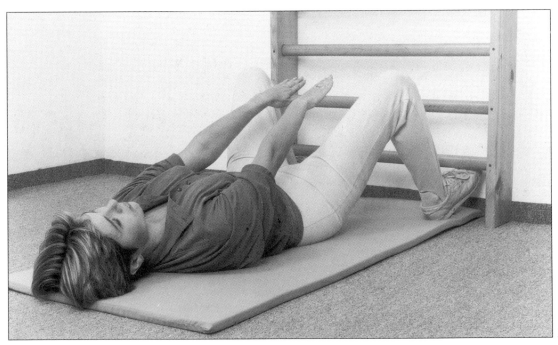

A

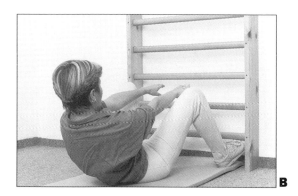

B

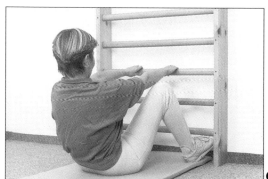

C

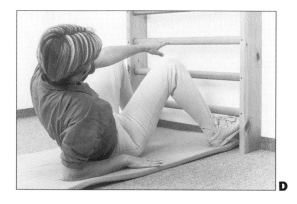

D

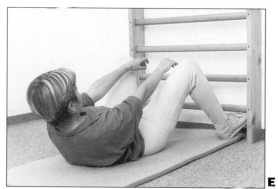

E

BACK/TUMMY 3

straight abdominal muscles

This exercise is very similar to the last one, except that you are working with a partner.

A Sit on floor facing your partner, your feet under his/her bent knees. Hold each other's wrists.

B Rotate pelvis back and lean back, pulling your partner towards you.

C Let go of his/her hands.

D Slowly roll your back flat on the floor counting 1, 2, 3.

E On the count of 4, lie flat with arms still outstretched. Rest for a few seconds. Talk to your partner.

F Now reverse the process, slowly curling your head and shoulders forward.

G Reach for your partner's hands.

H With partner's help, pull yourself back to start position A.

Repeat 15 times. Reverse roles and repeat another 15 times!

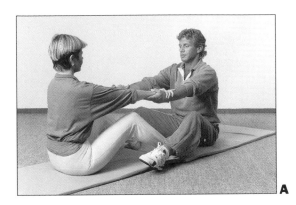

A

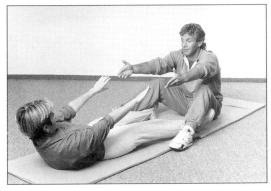

D

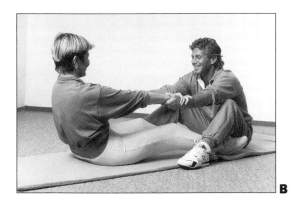

B

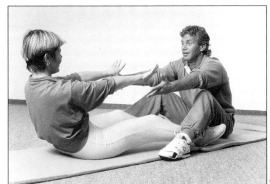

C

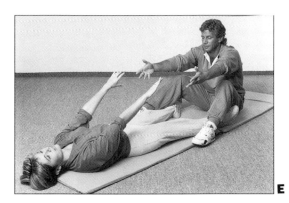

E

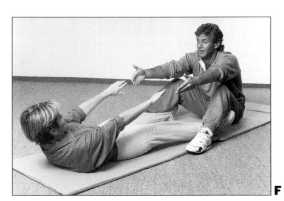

F

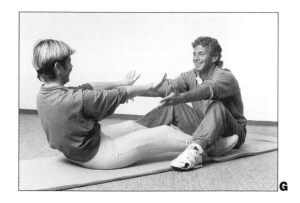

G

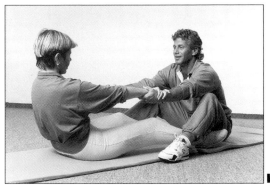

H

BACK/TUMMY 4

straight and oblique abdominal muscles

A Lie on back, knees shoulder-width apart and slightly bent, arms reaching forward.
B Lift head and shoulders and curl upper spine forwards, keeping lumbar spine flat on floor. Your hands should reach between your knees. Hold for 2 seconds, breathing naturally, then slowly uncurl and return to start position A. Repeat 10 times.
C With both arms stretched to right of right knee, curl upper spine towards right knee. Hold for 2 seconds, then uncurl and return to start position A. Repeat 10 times on each side.

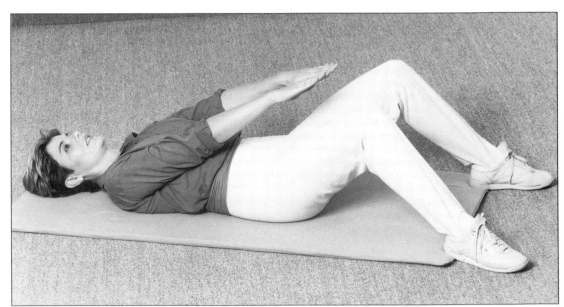

A

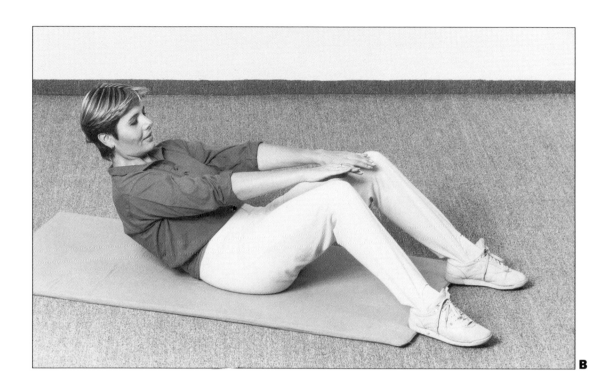

B

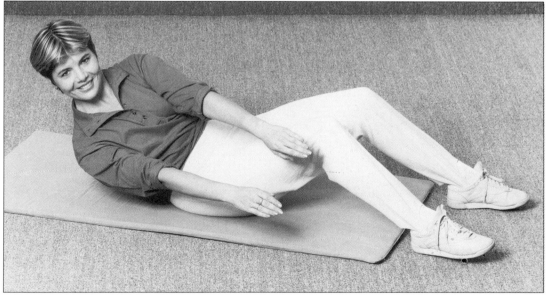

C

BACK/TUMMY 5

straight and oblique abdominals

This exercise also stretches the hamstrings, those (often tight) muscles at the back of the thighs.

A Lie on back with both legs straight and vertical, the right ankle in front of the left. Reach up with both arms.

B Curling head and shoulders off the floor, try to touch front ankle with fingertips. Hold for 3 seconds. Return to start position A. Repeat 10 times with the right ankle in front, and 10 times with the left ankle in front. Pause and hug knees.

C Now reach for the left side of your ankles with your right hand only. Hold for 3 seconds, return slowly to start position, and repeat with the other ankle in front.

D Repeat with opposite hand, changing ankles.

Repeat C and D 10 times. Pause and hug knees.

Finish by reaching up 5 times with both hands as in B.

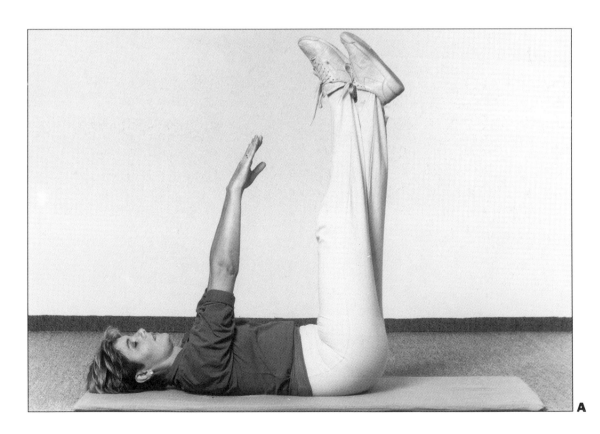

A

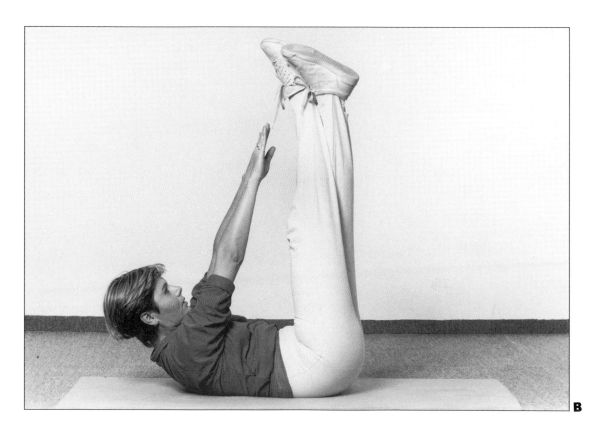

B

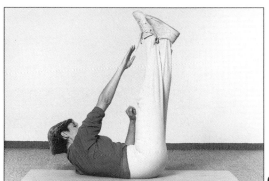

C

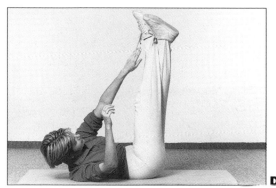

D

COOLING DOWN AND RELAXING

Cooling down is an important part of your workout, just as important as warming up. It allows your muscles to relax and your heart to slow down to its normal resting rhythm.

Cooling down should be enjoyable. You should enjoy the feeling of your body relaxing. A healthy person has the ability to relax properly, and not only after exercise. Without relaxation, how would we cope with the stresses and irritations of the modern world? In fact the routine outlined on the next few pages is a valuable anti-stress device. It takes only a minute or two and a little floor space.

COOL-DOWN 1

A Lie flat on back, legs slightly apart, arms loosely by sides, palms up.
B Tuck chin onto chest and press back of neck gently towards floor or into pillow.

Rotate your legs inward and outward. Point your toes hard, then relax, feeling the relaxation spread up your legs.
Roll your arms inward and outward. Clench and unclench your fists, and feel the relaxation spread up your arms.
Rotate your pelvis back a little, and feel your whole spine flatten and sink into the floor.

Close your eyes. Slowly roll your head from side to side a few times. Clench your teeth, then let your jaw drop and your lips part. Imagine gentle hands smoothing your forehead, cheeks and jaw.
Your breathing will become lighter and softer, and you will feel your body getting heavier. Be aware of the stillness and calm as your body loses its tensions. Let your mind become smooth and clear like the surface of a lake.
Stay in this relaxed state for at least 1 minute.

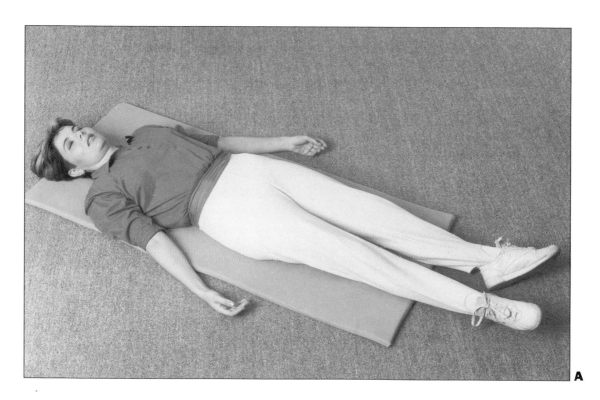

A

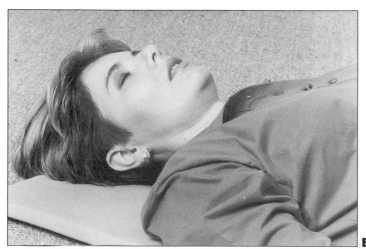

B

COOL-DOWN 2

A Roll over into a fetal position – on your side, arms and knees bent, head curled forward. Check your pulse.

B Push yourself up using your lower elbow and the palm of your other hand. Sit up, open your eyes, and smile to the world.

C Kneel on one knee, plant the other foot on the floor in front of you, and push yourself up into a standing position.

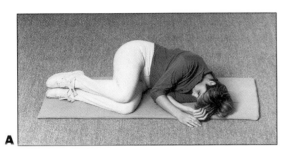

A

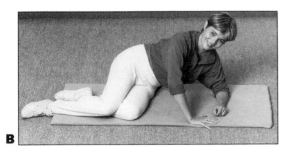

B

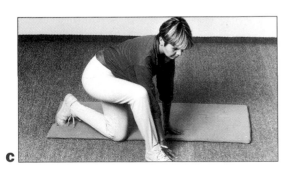

C

COOL-DOWN 3

A Stand sideways on to mirror, legs slightly apart, knees slightly bent, chin curled onto chest, arms loose by sides. Rotate your pelvis backward, tightening your buttocks and abdominal muscles.

B Slowly uncurl your spine – imagine it lengthening towards the ceiling, or imagine the vertebrae stacking one on top of the other like children's building blocks.

C Slightly de-rotate your pelvis, but continue to feel the pull of your abdominal muscles. Now balance your head and shoulders on top of your pelvis, lengthen the back of your neck and relax your shoulders down and back.

D Stand in this position for a few minutes, then turn and look at yourself in the mirror. This is the sort of posture you should always aim at – pelvis not tilted too far back or too far forward, buttocks relaxed, knees very slightly bent, upper body effortlessly balanced on top of the pelvis, neck long, chin level.

Walk slowly and smoothly about the room, keeping this new sense of looseness and balance. With perseverance, this will become your normal posture and your old posture will feel very odd.

Well, that's the end of your bone-loading workout. Congratulate yourself on having made and taken the time to do something good for yourself.

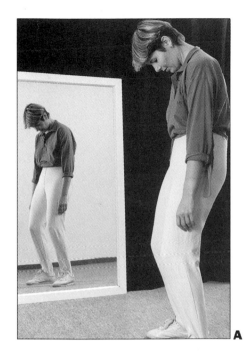

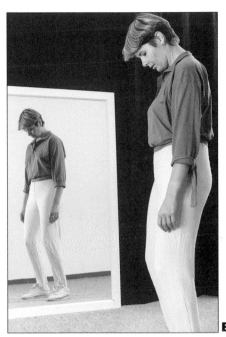

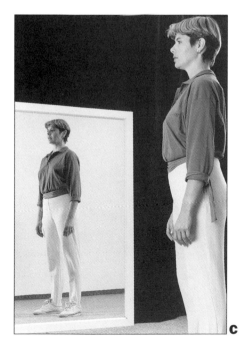

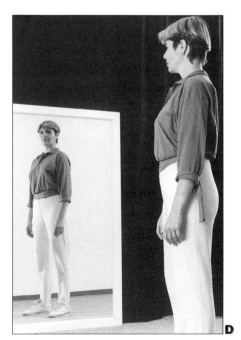

facts about

osteoporosis

**WHAT IS
OSTEOPOROSIS?**

Osteoporosis is progressive loss of bone density, a reduction of mass per unit volume. Over the years, as the result of slow depletion of bone substance, bone becomes increasingly porous, full of holes like a sponge, hence the name "osteo-porosis". The external shape and volume of the bones is not usually affected, but the internal structure becomes weaker, more fragile, more vulnerable to fracture and collapse. In elderly women with osteoporotic bones it is often the neck of the femur, the top part of the thigh bone, which eventually gives way.

This slow diminution of bone density occurs in men as well as women and is part of the natural and normal process of aging. By the age of 30 most of us have all the bone we are ever going to have. After that, bone density begins to decrease, at the rate of about 3 percent *per decade*. This means that most men, if they lead a fairly active life and are not in one of the risk categories listed on page 120, will arrive at the age of 80 with about 15 percent less bone than they had when they were 30. This is a significant loss, but not normally enough to cause bones to fracture during ordinary, everyday activities.

In women, the rate of bone loss accelerates after the menopause, which for most women is around the age of 50. For the next ten years or so bone may be lost at a rate of more than 3 percent *per year*. After that the rate of loss slows down. But by the time a woman is 60 she may have lost a substantial portion of bone from vital parts of her skeleton.

Bone loss is a hidden, silent process. It gives no pain or symptoms in its early stages. Then, without warning, a bone breaks, perhaps as a result of a minor stumble. A woman puts her arm out to prevent herself falling and breaks her radius, the bone on the thumb side of the forearm. Radius fractures are quite common in women aged 50–60. The bone usually breaks near the wrist, causing considerable pain because many muscles and ligaments are wrenched in the process, but after a few weeks in plaster it knits together fairly well, leaving wrist and forearm movements a little restricted but otherwise satisfactory.

Above the age of 60 fractures of the hip or upper part of the femur are more common. Steady loss of bone in this area, the neck of the femur, weakens the bone to such an extent that fracturing may be spontaneous, not the result of anything as forceful as a fall or a blow but simply a consequence of body weight or muscle

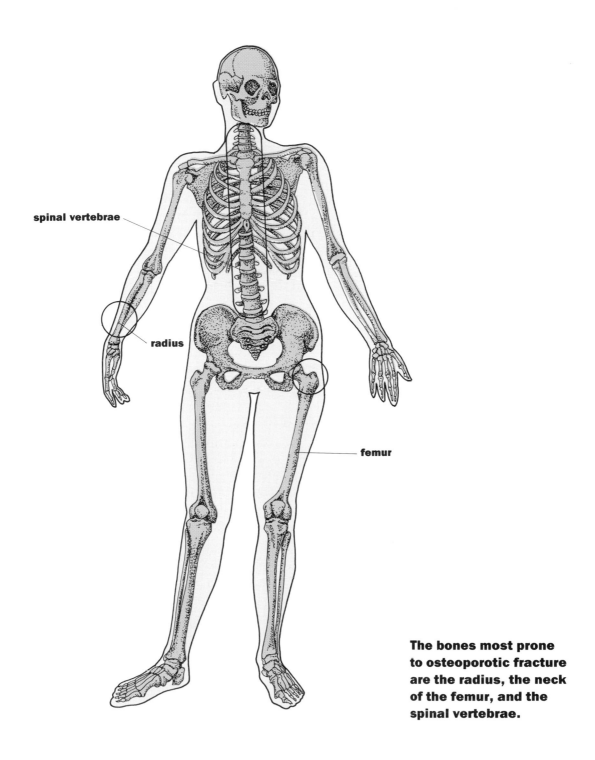

spinal vertebrae

radius

femur

The bones most prone to osteoporotic fracture are the radius, the neck of the femur, and the spinal vertebrae.

action. Hip fractures are potentially serious. First of all, they have to be "reduced" or realigned surgically, which involves several weeks in hospital. During convalescence, mobility is limited, which has adverse effects on almost all body systems, including the skeleton, heart and blood vessels. It may be many months before normal walking can be resumed. Because of the age at which hip fractures usually occur, typically after 70, general health is often poor and complications during and after the operation are common. The mortality rate among elderly women who break their hips is 12 percent during the year following the accident.

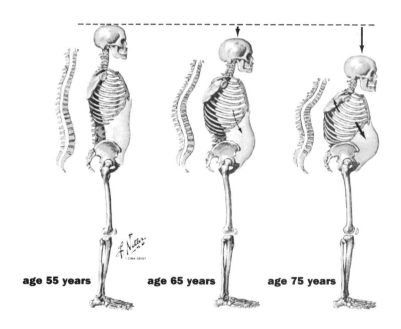

age 55 years   age 65 years   age 75 years

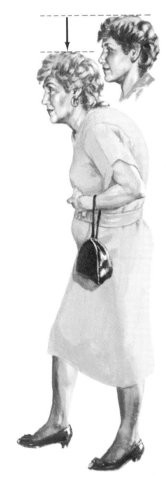

Changes in the spine and in posture due to osteoporosis of the spine. The dorsal vertebrae in particular, those between the neck and the waist, are prone to collapse. As the ribcage descends, the contents of the abdomen are compressed and pushed forwards.

The bones of the back, the spinal vertebrae, are also susceptible to osteoporosis. They are continually subjected to the compressive forces of body weight. As they weaken, small cracks appear in them, and they start to compress and distort. This results in a loss of height of 4 or 5 centimetres (about 2 inches) per decade and in the appearance of a hump or hunch back. The process may continue until the lower ribs actually lean on the top of the pelvis; by this time stature may have shortened by as much as 15–20 centimetres (6–8 inches). Spinal osteoporosis is quite common among elderly women. At the age of 70, about 25 percent of women have cracks in their vertebrae. Cracking of the vertebrae is often, although not invariably, accompanied by back pain.

The fact that there are several distinct types of osteoporotic fracture which tend to appear in two distinct age ranges has led some investigators to suggest that there are two different types of osteoporosis. One is "postmenopausal osteoporosis", which is peculiar to women. It causes accelerated bone loss after the menopause and fractures of the radius and spinal vertebrae. The other is "senile osteoporosis", or age-related bone loss. This is the slower, ongoing process which causes hip fractures – and a high incidence of other fractures as well – in both men and women of advanced years.

WHO IS AT RISK?

A risk factor is a habit, condition or set of circumstances which predisposes a person to develop a given disorder. In insidious disorders like osteoporosis, which may be symptomless for many years, it is especially important to know what the risk factors are. The most common are listed below. Unfortunately, it is not possible to assign a "weight" to each of these risks, since their relative importance varies from person to person. Nevertheless, if you are female, thin-boned, and appreciably below normal body weight for your build, you should regard yourself as being at risk. Lack of estrogen after the menopause increases that risk.

Because of the increased rate of bone loss after the menopause, many authorities recommend that all women should have their bone status measured at around the age of 50, with regular check-ups thereafter. There are various painless, non-invasive ways of doing this, as outlined on pages 128–132.

RISK FACTORS FOR OSTEOPOROSIS

AGE	Incidence and severity of osteoporosis increase with age.
SEX	For a decade or so after the menopause, women lose bone mass at a greater rate than men; fractures due to osteoporosis are more common in women than in men.
ETHNIC GROUP	Osteoporosis is more common among white, fair-haired people.
FAMILY HISTORY	The risk of osteoporosis increases if a close relative is/has been a sufferer.
EARLY MENOPAUSE	The earlier the menopause, the greater the risk of osteoporosis.
SKINNY BODY	Lean people with thin bones are more susceptible to osteoporosis than people of normal or heavy build.
OTHER DISORDERS	Osteoporosis may be secondary to a number of endocrine and metabolic disorders.
DRUGS	Osteoporosis can be caused by prolonged use of certain drugs, notably corticosteroids.
LACK OF EXERCISE	If bones are not regularly subjected to mechanical loading, "disuse osteoporosis" sets in.
LACK OF CALCIUM	Low reserves of bone can be the result of low calcium intake in childhood/adolescence.
LACK OF VITAMIN D	Lack of sunshine or lack of dietary vitamin D hampers absorption of calcium from the gut.
ALCOHOL, TOBACCO, CAFFEINE, ANIMAL PROTEIN	Osteoporosis seems to be linked with excessive consumption of these.

Risk factors which cannot be avoided

Age and sex Bone loss begins during the fourth decade of life, after the age of 30. As each decade passes, the signs and symptoms of osteoporosis – fractures, back pain, loss of height, rounded back – become more and more likely. But at all ages, women are four or five times more likely to suffer from osteoporotic fractures than men. This is because, after the menopause, the ovaries no longer produce the female sex hormone estrogen. In women, estrogen is the single most important guardian of bone mass.

Ethnic group Surveys conducted in several continents have shown that osteoporosis is more common among Caucasians and Orientals than among people of African origin.

Family history There seems to be a hereditary component to rapid bone loss after the menopause. Women whose mothers or sisters suffer from osteoporosis seem to be more susceptible. Studies of identical twins have shown that genetic factors affect peak bone mass and its rate of decrease.

Risk factors which are partly controllable

Early menopause As we have seen, bone loss increases sharply for a few years after the menopause. This remains true whether the menopause occurs around the age of 50 or whether it occurs earlier, after surgical removal of the ovaries for example. As a rule, the earlier the menopause, the more likely a woman is to suffer from osteoporosis. When the uterus is removed without removing the ovaries, menstruation ceases but bone mass is not affected because the ovaries are still active. The main hormone produced by the ovaries is estrogen. Lack of this hormone is perhaps the most important single cause of osteoporosis in women, even though the mechanism by which it influences bone formation or destruction is not known. Any woman who has had a hysterectomy should find out if her ovaries were removed during the operation.

An early menopause, at or below the age of 45, can be quite spontaneous or it may be a symptom of some other condition, in which case medical advice should be sought.

Skinny body Various researchers have found that women with small, thin bones are more susceptible to osteoporotic fractures than women of sturdier build. The reason for this may be that they have less peak bone mass to start with, smaller reserves on which to draw when the process of bone loss begins. Their bones therefore weaken earlier. Also, since small quantities of female hormones are produced in fatty tissue even when the ovaries are no longer active, women of heavier build still have some estrogen after the menopause, which may protect them to some extent against rapid bone loss. Skinny women do not have these reserves of fat. In addition, the higher body weight of heavier women also serves as a constant mechanical load on their bones, which may have a beneficial effect on bone growth. Fatty tissue is also a shock absorber, padding the body against impact and reducing the risk of fracture.

This does not mean that putting on weight is recommended as a way of preventing osteoporosis. Being overweight has, as we all know, serious drawbacks – among other things, it overtaxes the heart, the circulation and the joints. However, deliberate and exaggerated weight reduction should be avoided as it can disrupt the function of the ovaries. Anorexia nervosa causes infertility as well as general damage to the heart, liver and kidneys.

Other disorders Osteoporosis is sometimes secondary to other disorders which directly or indirectly affect the whole metabolism of the body. If the underlying cause is correctly diagnosed and treated, the osteoporotic process can usually be halted or reversed. Conditions which cause osteoporosis include hyperactivity of the thyroid or parathyroid glands, chronic renal failure and diabetes mellitus. Of special interest are conditions which affect the secretion of sex hormones in men. Men have no ovaries and no menopause, so the main cause of osteoporosis in women, the withdrawal of estrogen, does not apply. Nevertheless even in young men decreased testicular hormonal activity (hypogonadism) can lead to osteoporosis. Osteoporosis associated with alcoholism is also thought to be due to reduced levels of male sex hormone. Some malabsorption syndromes (conditions in which food is poorly absorbed from the gut) and certain tumors can also cause osteoporosis.

Drugs The drugs most commonly implicated in the development of osteoporosis are the corticosteroids, used for their anti-inflammatory, anti-allergic and anti-rheumatic effects. Unfortunately their side-effects are not at all useful. Doctors are aware of this and only prescribe them when there is no alternative. The effect of cortisone on bone can be minimized, although not eliminated, by giving supplements of vitamin D and calcium.

It should also be borne in mind that diuretics and laxatives increase calcium losses in the urine and feces.

Risk factors which can be eliminated

Lack of physical activity Time and time again, research has shown that enforced or obligatory inactivity causes the kind of bone loss known as "disuse osteoporosis" or "immobilization osteoporosis". Enforced inactivity can be the result of prolonged bed rest or several weeks in a spacecraft, but a sedentary lifestyle has similar though less rapid and drastic effects. Unfortunately most people in the Western world are not as physically active on a regular daily basis as they should be. The effects of physical activity on bone growth are discussed on page 132.

Lack of calcium in the diet Calcium salts are the main component of bone tissue – with phosphate, they give bone its structural strength. Although low calcium intake over a long period encourages the osteoporotic process, lack of calcium alone is not the cause of osteoporosis. Simply adding calcium to the diet does not cure or prevent it. Nevertheless, most experts agree that an adequate daily intake of calcium is necessary throughout life to prevent bone loss. The role of calcium in relation to osteoporosis is discussed on page 138.

Alcohol, tobacco, caffeine, animal protein A number of studies have shown that hip fractures are more common in male and female alcoholics than in their non-alcoholic peers. Women who smoke tend to reach the menopause earlier than non-smoking women, which predisposes them to earlier signs of osteoporosis. Nicotine is an estrogen antagonist. However, at the moment there is no clear concensus as to whether smoking *per se* increases the risk of osteoporosis. Excessive consumption of caffeine, found in tea, cocoa, chocolates and cola drinks as well as coffee, is also thought to be a contributory factor. There also seems to be a correlation between osteoporosis and the consumption of large amounts of animal protein.

Now that you are familiar with some of the consequences of and reasons for bone loss, you may be curious to know a little more about bones themselves.

There is a beauty and elegance about the internal structure of bone which is not seen by the naked eye. At first sight, bone appears hard, lifeless, a dull but necessary material to which tendons and ligaments are attached. As a matter of fact, bone is as complex, dynamic and active as any other tissue of the body.

Bone is one of the last tissues to appear during fetal development. At birth most of a baby's bones are still made of cartilage, which is soft and flexible, although it contains small "ossification centers" from which bone gradually spreads until it replaces the cartilage completely. Throughout life, from babyhood to old age, bone undergoes a continuous process of reconstruction, reshaping and reorganization. This is how worn-out bone is replaced with new bone and how fractures heal. Until the end of adolescence, that is until the age of 18–20, this constant remodeling process is part of general body growth. Between 20 and 30, the bones continue to grow, although they do not increase in length; they become wider and thicker instead. At age 30, peak bone mass is reached. Thereafter, as we have seen, bone is slowly lost. But even into old age the internal remodeling and renewal process goes on, although at a slower pace.

Bone is almost immortal. It can survive, almost unchanged, for thousands of years. This is because a large part of it, about 65 percent, consists of an inorganic material called hydroxyapatite, a salt of calcium and phosphorus. The other 35 percent is organic and consists mainly of a fibrous protein called collagen. Collagen is the main building material of all the other "connective" tissues of the body – skin, cartilage, tendons, ligaments, fascia. The word collagen is, most appropriately, derived from the Greek word *kolla* meaning "glue". At one time, glue made from animal bones was used extensively in the furniture industry. Now it has been replaced by synthetic plastic adhesives.

The thin fibers of collagen, less than one thousandth of a millimeter thick, are reinforced by still thinner crystals of hydroxyapatite. The reinforced fibers are organized into bundles, and the bundles are organized into elaborate three-dimensional structures designed to withstand the mechanical loads exerted by gravity, the pull of muscles, and impact. This structure makes bone one of the most economical building materials in nature.

If you look at a longitudinal section through a long bone, one of the limb bones for example, you will see that it looks like a hollow tube. The wall of the tube is made of compact bone a few millimeters thick. This dense outer layer of bone is referred to as

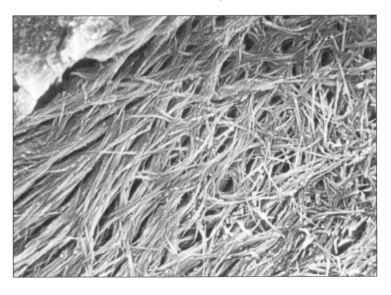

Bundles of collagen fibers in bone, magnified many times under an electron microscope.

"compact bone". The space in the center of the tube is filled with a soft, semi-liquid substance. This is bone marrow, the very active tissue that specializes in producing new blood cells and exporting them through the blood to all parts of the body.

Towards the two ends of the bone, the wall of the tube becomes thinner, perhaps as thin as 1 millimeter, and the space inside is occupied by a different kind of bone. This is made of the same material as compact bone – fibres of collagen reinforced with crystals of hydroxyapatite – but it has a looser, meshlike structure. The bony struts which make up the mesh are called "trabeculae", a Latin word meaning "scaffolding". The spaces between the trabeculae are filled with bone marrow. This type of bone is known as "trabecular", "spongy" or "cancellous" bone. The bodies of the spinal vertebrae are made of spongy bone surrounded by a thin layer of compact bone.

Compact and trabecular bone are masterpieces of mechanical engineering, but they are not alive. Life is given to them by numerous cells called "osteocytes" dispersed throughout their

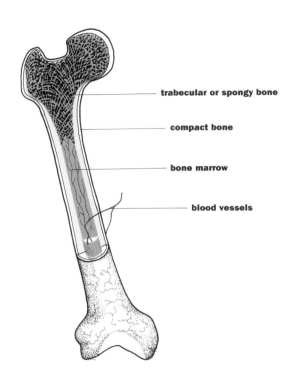

trabecular or spongy bone

compact bone

bone marrow

blood vessels

A longitudinal section through a normal femur, showing the tubular structure of long bones and the spongy, honeycomb-like structure of bone at their ends. The spinal vertebrae are completely filled with spongy bone.

structure. These cells swap small amounts of calcium between bone and blood in order to keep the calcium in the blood at a constant level. They are interconnected by a network of thin cytoplasmic extensions which lie in tiny channels called "canaliculi." Compact bone is also threaded by another network of channels containing small blood vessels. These supply the osteocytes with oxygen and nutrients, and are also the route by which other types of cells, those concerned with bone breakdown and bone renewal, migrate to almost every part of compact bone. In spongy bone, exchanges between blood and osteocytes are even easier because the trabeculae are filled with bone marrow.

Bone renewal is achieved by a process of remodeling in which old bone has to be broken down before new bone can take its place. This process is performed by the orchestrated action of two populations of cells, destroyers and builders. The destroyers, or "osteoclasts", appear first and start to break down and engulf small areas of calcified collagen, widening existing holes within it. Within a few days they have created a cylindrical hole. Then a group of builder cells, or osteoblasts, appears and starts depositing layers of collagen within the hole. As the collagen starts to calcify and harden, the osteoblasts become trapped by their own handiwork. They then cease their building activities and become osteocytes.

What controls the numbers and levels of activity of osteoblasts and osteoclasts? Two hormones, principally, calci-

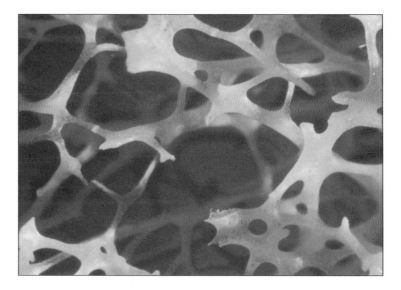

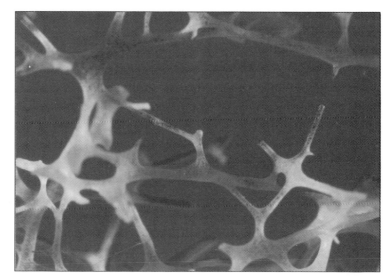

In normal trabecular bone (above) there are many bony struts. In osteoporotic bone (below) there are fewer and thinner struts. Trabecular bone is lost at a greater rate than compact bone.

tonin produced by the thyroid gland and parathyroid hormone produced by the four parathyroid glands embedded in the back of the thyroid gland. Calcitonin depresses osteoclast activity and parathyroid hormone promotes it. Vitamin D enhances the effects of calcitonin and estrogen seems to make osteoclasts less sensitive to parathyroid hormone.

Bone remodeling is a normal process which goes on throughout life. During childhood and adolescence it ensures that the lengthwise growth of bones keeps pace with their increase in girth; if it did not, their proportions would be all wrong. In adulthood it ensures that old, fatigued bone tissue is replaced with new. And throughout life remodeling enables our bones to adapt to the mechanical forces which act on them, adding bone to regions where load is high and removing it from places where load is small or non-existent.

It is precisely because bone has the potential to renew itself in response to mechanical forces that bone-loading physical exercise offers such hope in the prevention and treatment of osteoporosis. In women and men affected by osteoporosis the equilibrium between the destructive activity of osteoclasts and the constructive activity of osteoblasts is disturbed, and the scales tip towards the side of net bone loss. Exactly how this balance becomes disturbed is not known. Various factors seem to play a part – hormones, diet, physical activity, lifestyle. The available treatments, discussed on pages 147–151, all aim to alter one or other of these factors in a positive direction.

HOW IS BONE LOSS MEASURED?

Until about 10 years ago the only means of evaluating loss of bone mass was by radiography, or X-ray. But bone loss does not show up on an X-ray until the bones concerned have lost 30–40 percent of their mass. X-rays are not sensitive enough to detect smaller changes in bone density. To ensure earlier detection and treatment, and in order to assess the effects of exercise, diet, drugs and hormones on the process of bone loss, better diagnostic methods had to be developed.

Today there are several accurate methods of measuring bone status. These enable bone loss to be detected early and its progress monitored. The bones most commonly measured, because they are the ones most susceptible to osteoporotic weakening, are those in the forearm (radius and ulna), the thigh bone near the hip joint (neck of the femur), and the spinal vertebrae. The measuring process involves exposing the bones to small doses of radiation, and the results are accurate to within 2–5 percent.

Single photon absorptiometry (SPA) This is the oldest of the modern methods. The bone in question – usually the distal part of the radius, the wrist end of the radius – is scanned crosswise with a ray of photons or light particles emitted by a radioactive source, usually radioactive iodine. The larger the amount of calcium in

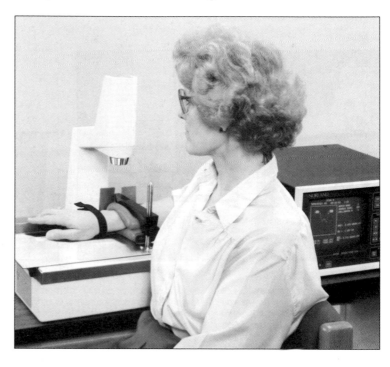

In this picture bone mineral content of the forearm is being methods by the Single Photon Absorptiometry method. Note the water-filled cuff around the lower forearm.

the way of the photons, the smaller the number of photons which pass through the bone. Those which do pass through are "counted" by a radiation meter. The soft tissues around the bone – skin, muscles, fat – absorb some radiation, so it is important to ensure that the photons are always directed at the same total thickness of tissue. To even out the differences in soft tissue thickness as the forearm tapers towards the wrist, the forearm is wrapped in a cuff containing water.

An SPA scan of part of the forearm takes about five minutes and the results, expressed in grams of minerals per square centimeter of bone, are displayed on a computer screen.

How, you may ask, can the spine or the hip bone be wrapped in water in order to do an SPA scan? The answer is, they can't. To measure bone density in these areas another method has to be used.

Dual Photo Absorptiometry (DPA) This method is similar to the one above but can be used to measure the mineral content of the vertebrae and the neck of the femur, and of other bones if necessary. Because the radioactive source emits photons in two distinct energy bands, it is possible to calculate the effect of soft tissues on photon absorption.

Dual Photon X-ray can be used to measure the mineral content of any bone. Here it is being used to assess the status of the lower back, or lumbar, vertebrae. The legs are raised to allow the lumbar curve to flatten.

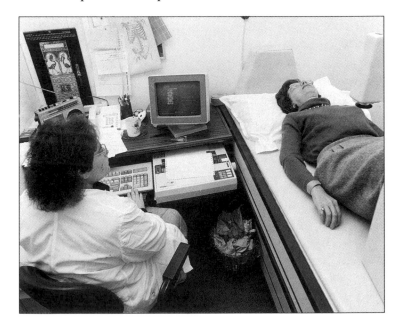

A new version of this method, Dual Photon X-ray (DPX), has been introduced recently. The light source in this case is not a radioactive element like iodine but an X-ray tube. DPX is both quicker and more accurate than DPA.

A DPA or DPX scan takes between 10 and 20 minutes.

Computed Tomography (CT) The disadvantage of the methods mentioned so far is that they cannot distinguish between compact bone and spongy bone. This is important, since bone loss begins in trabecular bone. Computed tomography enables the density of both types of bone to be measured separately.

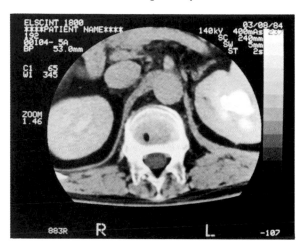

A CT scan of a lumbar vertebra, viewed from beneath.

CT scanning was introduced about 20 years ago and it has brought about a revolution in X-ray diagnosis. With this method, a thin beam of X-rays is sent into the body and a small detector on the opposite side of the body measures the amount of radiation which passes through. This procedure is repeated many times, each time with the X-ray beam rotated slightly in relation to the body. The resulting image is a composite of all the sections scanned by the beam, showing all the tissues in the particular cross-section or slice of the body through which the beam has passed. Each tissue absorbs the X-ray beam differently, depending on its density and chemical composition. So with a CT scan one can measure bone density at any point within the body provided its chemical composition is known.

The difficulty is that the chemical composition of bone differs in different people, and even in different parts of the body. This can be overcome by using two wavelengths of X-rays, but this doubles the amount of radiation used, which is already comparatively high. CT apparatus is also extremely expensive.

131

Compton Spectrometry This method was developed at the Physics Institute of the Hebrew University in Jerusalem, in collaboration with the Jerusalem Osteoporosis Center of the Hadassah University Hospital. It enables bone density (grams of bone per cubic centimeter) to be measured in almost any part of the skeleton. Like CT, it distinguishes between compact and spongy bone, but unlike CT it does not depend on the chemical composition of the bone being measured.

The method is based on a phenomenon known as the Compton effect: when a material is exposed to a beam of high energy photons, the photons which are not absorbed are scattered in different directions and the number of photons scattered in a direction perpendicular to the beam at a given point is proportional to the density of the material at that point.

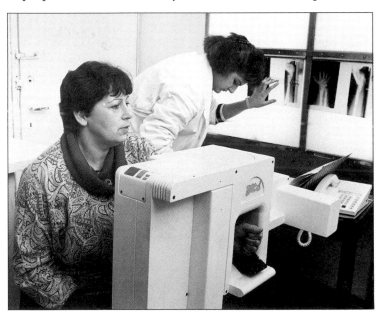

Bone density can be measured directly by Compton Spectrometry. This instrument uses radioactive caesium (Cs-137) as its photon source.

WHY DOES BONE-LOADING INCREASE BONE DENSITY?

Living bones adapt themselves, both in size and internal structure, to the mechanical forces applied to them. This relationship, between bone morphology and applied forces, was first noticed by Galileo in 1683. In 1892 the German anatomist Julius Wolff observed: "Every change in the function of a bone is followed by certain definite changes in internal architecture. . . ."

If an increase in load causes an increase in bone mass, the converse is also true. People who are bedridden for long periods rapidly lose bone mass. The bone of a paralyzed limb loses mass. The bone of a limb immobilized in a plaster cast loses mass. The bones of astronauts living in space lose mass – there is no gravity to compress, bend, twist and stretch them. The astronauts aboard Skylab lost calcium from their bones at the astonishing rate of 200 mg per day. However, disuse osteoporosis is a reversible process. Bone mass is regained when regular physical activity is resumed, although the rate at which this happens is much slower than the rate at which bone was lost.

Conversely, people who habitually engage in intense physical activity – lumberjacks and athletes, for example – have thicker, heavier bones than non-active people of the same age. One study, for example, found that total body calcium in a group of marathon runners (mean age 42) was 7 percent higher than that in a control group.

Only those bones which are subjected to intense and repeated loading increase in mass. The effect is very specific. Thus, a right-handed tennis player will have thicker, heavier bones in his right arm than in his left. Nevertheless, someone who maintains a high level of activity for many years is likely to have a high bone mass in later life, higher than average for his or her age. A high level of mechanical usage over an extended period causes an accumulation of bone mass. This mass is rather like a savings account, a line of credit to be drawn upon when, due to declining physical and hormonal activity, bone destruction begins to outstrip bone building.

This raises two important questions. First, is it possible to increase bone mass in someone who is already old? Second, can controlled physical activity increase bone mass by a significant amount, or at least prevent further loss, in people who do not regularly engage in strenuous exercise? Before we try to answer these questions, let us look at some recent research in this field.

In the last decade there have been several animal studies which set out to investigate the relationship between various mechanical forces acting on bone and the rate and location of bone gain. As in so many other fields, animal experiments have enabled researchers to do work which could not have been done with people. This is what they found:

The effect of mechanical force is local. Bone mass only increases in those bones which are subjected to load.

The rate at which bone is gained depends on the magnitude of the force applied to it and on the speed with which that force is applied. The higher the load and the more swiftly is it applied, the greater the rate of bone gain. Beyond a certain level and rate of load, of course, bones break, so it is important to work within physiological limits.

To achieve a steady, sustained rate of bone gain, force must be applied repeatedly on a daily basis. The number of repetitions required per day is not particularly high – between 10 and 30 – but beyond that number loading ceases to be effective.

A variety of mechanical forces must be applied, particularly those which impose "unusual" forces on bone, forces which are not part of normal activity patterns.

This issue of diversity of forces is important. All objects, including bones, can be stretched, compressed, bent or twisted – engineers refer to these forces as tension, compression, bending and torsion – or they can be subjected to a combination of these forces. The direction in which these forces act on the bone can be applied in an unusual direction. For instance, the femur can be bent in a fore-and-aft direction (in the "sagittal" plane) or sideways (in the "coronal" plane), or it can be twisted clockwise or counterclockwise. During habitual activities, such as walking, compressive forces are certainly exerted on the femur, but no diversity of loading is achieved.

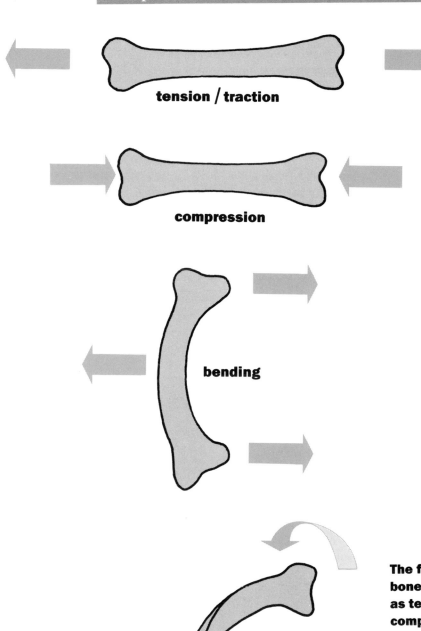

tension / traction

compression

bending

torsion

The forces which act on bones can be classified as tension, compression, bending or torsion, or as combinations of these. Unusual loads are those most valuable in increasing bone density.

Key experiment

With the knowledge gained from working with animals, researchers felt more confident about applying that knowledge to people. In 1985 the authors and several colleagues working at the Hebrew University and Haddassah Medical Organization in Jerusalem decided to try to find answers to the following questions: Could a set of exercises be designed which exerted diverse, dynamic forces on living human bone? Could such exercises be made suitable for middle-aged and older women? Would such exercises, if done regularly and systematically, increase bone mass? And if so, by how much?

In order to answer these questions we asked a group of fourteen women to take part in an experimental bone-loading program for a period of five months. The youngest woman was 53 and the oldest 74, and all of them were diagnosed as having mild osteoporosis. The bone-loading program consisted of three weekly sessions of 50 minutes each. About 20 minutes of each session were devoted to bone-loading exercises for the forearms, exercises which exerted tension, compression, bending and torsion. During the rest of the session the group did warm-up, flexibility and cool-down exercises, and exercises to strengthen the back and the abdominal muscles. A second group of twenty-six women, of similar age and also diagnosed as having mild osteoporosis, served as a control group. They did not take part in the bone-loading program. Neither they nor the women in the bone-loading group were physically active before the experiment.

Each woman in both groups had the density of bone in her distal radius measured on three separate occasions, one year before the bone-loading program started, at the beginning of the program, and at the end of the program. The method used was the Compton scattering technique described on page 132. The results are shown in the graph below.

During the year leading up to the program, mean bone density in both groups of women diminished by 2–3 percent. By the end of the program mean bone density in the control group had dwindled by a further 2 percent, but that of the bone-loading group had increased by nearly 4 percent. A 4 percent gain may not sound much, but it effectively restored the radii of the women concerned to the status they had 12–18 months earlier. What is more, complaints of back pain significantly decreased. The women in both groups were asked to grade their back pain before and after the program, and while there was no change in the level of complaints of back pain in the control group, there was a clear improvement in the exercise group. No damage to bones, joints or muscles was found during or at the end of the exercise period.

This graph shows the results of the Jerusalem study. Whereas density of the radius increased by nearly 4 percent in the bone-loading group, in the control group it continued to decrease.

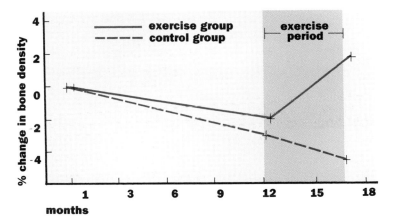

Similar studies carried out in the United States, Canada, United Kingdom and Denmark have produced similar results. This is very encouraging. It is possible, with suitable physical activity, to improve bone status in postmenopausal women. And even women unused to exercise do not find such activity hard or difficult, provided it is done carefully, gradually and under professional supervision.

However, in follow-up studies it has been found that bone mass returns to pre-exercise levels if exercise is not continued. This was the case in one study which measured bone mass six months after exercise stopped, and in another which measured bone mass after one year. This points to a very important fact: bone-loading exercises are not a short-term, once-only form of treatment for osteoporosis. They should become a regular, lifelong habit. In the authors' experience, and in the experience of other pioneers of bone-loading, it can quickly become an enjoyable habit, especially if done with a partner or in a group. That is why we very much hope that the exercises and information in this book will be adopted by those who run exercise and keep-fit classes.

As always, certain warnings should be sounded. In the advanced stages of osteoporosis, extra loading of bones may precipitate fractures. Anyone who belongs to two or more of the risk categories mentioned on page 120 should seek medical advice before embarking on a bone-loading program.

Physical activity may also be damaging to older people for reasons which have nothing to do with the status of their bones — they may have heart disease, high blood pressure, or arthritis, for example. Anyone over the age of 40 who is unaccustomed to physical exercise but wants to start exercising should see his or her GP and ask for a check-up.

HOW DOES DIET AFFECT BONES?

We have already seen that about two-thirds of bone tissue is made of a calcium mineral, hydroxyapatite. Adequate calcium in the diet is therefore important in early life, when bone is growing fastest, but it is also important in later life when it can help to prevent decay.

Calcium

Calcium is the most abundant mineral in the human body. A man's body contains 950–1,300 grams (2⅛–2¾ lbs) of calcium, depending on his height and build, and a woman's 770–920 grams (1¾–2 lbs). Ninety-nine percent of this is stored in the bones and teeth, giving them their hardness and structural strength. Although the amount of calcium elsewhere in the body — in the blood, other body fluids, and in soft tissues — is very small, it is absolutely critical to such functions as muscle contraction, nerve conduction, blood clotting and many other chemical processes.

The level of calcium in the blood is kept within very narrow limits by an elaborate hormonal and biochemical control system. Small quantities of calcium are continually swapped between the bones and the blood in order to keep the level of calcium in the blood constant. Any excess is usually lost in the feces, urine and sweat.

Food is the body's only source of calcium. Typically, we consume about 800 mg of calcium a day, but within 24 hours, if our hormonal and biochemical control system is working properly, we will also have lost 800 mg. The amount of calcium entering the body therefore equals the amount that leaves it, and the amount of calcium in the skeleton remains constant. The diagram below shows how "zero calcium balance" is achieved.

What happens if we increase our daily intake of calcium? More calcium will be lost in the feces, urine and sweat, so the net

Calcium absorption in the gut is not particularly efficient even in a young healthy adult. Only half of it is absorbed, and the same amount is lost in the urine, sweat and digestive juices. In this way calcium in the blood and bones remains constant.

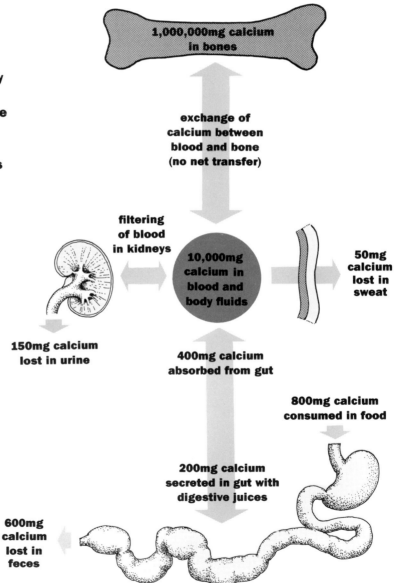

1,000,000mg calcium in bones

exchange of calcium between blood and bone (no net transfer)

filtering of blood in kidneys

10,000mg calcium in blood and body fluids

50mg calcium lost in sweat

150mg calcium lost in urine

400mg calcium absorbed from gut

800mg calcium consumed in food

200mg calcium secreted in gut with digestive juices

600mg calcium lost in feces

139

calcium balance remains the same, zero. This balance will only shift to the positive side if more calcium is absorbed from the intestines. Then, given sufficient physical activity and the right mix of hormones, more calcium will be laid down in the bones.

How much calcium do we need?

This depends on age, sex, weight and the way in which our body deals with calcium. Every few years a committee of the American Academy of Science updates the Recommended Dietary Allowances (RDAs) of various foods, and the most recent RDAs for calcium for various groups are given below.

CALCIUM
Recommended Dietary Allowance in mg per day

up to 6 months	360
6–12 months	540
1–10 years	800
10–18 years	1,200
18–50 years	800
during pregnancy and	1,600 mothers under 19
breast-feeding	1,200 mothers over 19
women over 50	1,000–1,500
men and women over 60	1,000–1,500

Children and adolescents Most of the calcium in an adult's body is accumulated between birth and the age of 18–20. Total accumulation during this period is of the order of 1,000–1,200 grams, acquired at the rate of 140–180 mg per day. Growth is most rapid between 10 and 18 – during this time we acquire 45 percent of our adult bone mass, accumulating bone at the rate of 250–500 mg per day. In girls, growth is fastest at around the age of 12; in boys maximum rate of growth occurs about two years later.

Younger children also grow rapidly, but their total body mass is smaller and so their calcium requirements are also smaller. The RDA for children aged 1–10 years is 800 mg per day. For children aged 6–12 months it is 540 mg per day, and for the first six months it is 360 mg per day.

Young adults After adolescence, our bones cease to grow in length, but until the age of 30 they continue to increase in thickness. The bone mass which accumulates during this period tops up the bone mass acquired by the age of 18–20, and becomes the reserve on which we draw throughout the rest of our lives. When our calcium balance becomes negative, bone loss begins, so it is extremely important to consume sufficient calcium between the age of 20 and 30. The RDA for this age group is 800 mg per day, although some researchers recommend 1,000 mg.

During pregnancy and breast-feeding Calcium requirements increase during the second half of pregnancy and during breast-feeding. For mothers of 19 or older, the RDA is 1,200 mg per day. For younger mothers it is 1,600 mg.

After the menopause Bone loss is most rapid in the five years or so following the menopause. Increasing calcium consumption during this period is not sufficient to slow down the osteoporotic process, because at this age the main reason for bone loss is lack of estrogen. Nevertheless, women in their 50s should increase their RDA of calcium to 1,000–1,500 mg per day.

Although, bone loss in women slows down after the age of 60 or so, absorption of calcium from the gut becomes less efficient as we grow older. Many experts therefore recommend 1,000–1,500 mg per day for both men and women over 60.

WARNING Although excessive consumption of calcium for short periods has no adverse effect on a healthy adult, for someone with kidney or digestive tract disease high calcium consumption can cause calcium to be deposited in the kidneys and soft tissues. Such people should consult their GP before increasing their calcium intake.

Sources of calcium Animal and vegetable foods containing high levels of calcium are listed on pages 143–146. Their calorie content is also given, so that if you are weight-watching you can choose items which are high in calcium but relatively low in calories. Only foods which have a calcium content higher than 100 mg per 100 grams (3½ oz) have been included.

There is a catch, however, and that is that the amount of calcium the gut absorbs from foods containing identical amounts of calcium is not the same. The gut can only absorb calcium if it is in soluble form, and the extent to which the calcium in a particular food is soluble depends on the way it is linked to other substances in that food.

The use of calcium supplements to treat osteoporosis is briefly discussed on page 150.

Milk and milk products These are particularly rich in calcium. Since babies and all young mammals grow and thrive on milk it is hardly surprising that the calcium it contains is soluble or bound to casein, the main milk protein, and is therefore well absorbed. The only drawback with milk products is that some of them, hard cheeses in particular, are a concentrated source of saturated fatty acids, which are the kind of fatty acids the body stores rather than uses constructively. Fortunately low-fat dairy products contain just as much calcium, and sometimes more, than those high in fat.

Meat and fish Meat contains very little calcium, and in any case heavy consumption of animal protein increases the acidity of the urine and therefore increases the amount of calcium lost in the urine. Fish, especially small fish such as whitebait, sprats and sardines which are usually eaten with the bones, or canned salmon, mackerel or pilchards on the bone, contain appreciable amounts of calcium. Oysters and scallops are also a reasonable source.

Vegetables, pulses, seeds and nuts Calcium can be obtained solely from plant sources. However, since many plant foods also contain oxalic or phytic acid, which inhibits the absorption of calcium, a certain amount of knowledge is necessary to ensure an adequate daily intake. Anyone who is a strict vegetarian or allergic to milk products would do well to consult a nutritionist or buy a book on the subject. Interestingly, in people who regularly eat foods containing phytic acid (pulses, cereals), the body starts to produce an enzyme called phytase which breaks down phytic acid, allowing their calcium to be absorbed. Of course there are many plant foods, some of the herbs and spices for instance, and blackstrap molasses, which are very high in calcium but eaten in such small quantities that they cannot be regarded as useful sources. Cocoa beans, coffee beans and tea leaves also contain appreciable amounts of calcium, but the beverages prepared from them do not add significantly to calcium consumption; in fact they do the reverse, since the phytates they contain hinder absorption of calcium from the gut.

Fruit Generally speaking, fruit contains only a fraction of the calcium found in dairy foods and certain vegetables and seeds. Dried figs are the big exception. Raw blackberries, dried dates, raisins, raspberries and blackcurrants contain between a quarter and a third of the calcium of dried figs.

MILK
Calcium content and energy value

	Average calcium mg/100g	Energy kcal/100g
Cow's milk – whole milk	120	69
fat-reduced, 3.5% fat	120	67
fat-reduced, 1.5–1.8% fat	118	49
fat-reduced, 0.2–1.2% fat	123	35
Sheep's milk	183	100
Goat's milk	127	72

Human milk, by comparison, contains only 25–41 mg of calcium per 100g although its energy value, 71 kcal/100g, is similar to that of whole cow's milk.

MILK PRODUCTS
Calcium content and energy value

	Average calcium mg/100g	Energy kcal/100g
Condensed milk, 7.5% fat	242	137
Condensed milk, 10% fat	315	182
Condensed milk, sweetened	238	325
Condensed skimmed milk, sweetened	340	273
Whole milk powder	920	506
Skimmed milk powder	1,290	371
Cream, 10% fat	101	127
Cream, 30% fat	80	317
Sour cream, 18% fat	100	192
Yogurt, 3.5% fat	120	71
Yogurt, 1.5–1.8% fat	114	51
Yogurt, 0.3% fat	143	39
Milk chocolate	214	550

CHEESES
Calcium content and energy value

	Average calcium mg/100g	Energy kcal/100g
Bel Paese	604	391
Brie, 50% fat	400	358
Camembert, 30% fat	600	228
Camembert, 50% fat	510	328
Cheddar, 50% fat	810	410
Edam, 30% fat	800	266
Edam, 50% fat	678	371
Blue cheese	526	368
Emmenthal	1,020	401
Feta	429	260
Gorgonzola	612	374
Gouda, 45% fat	820	382
Gruyère	1,000	430
Limburger, 20% fat	510	195
Limburger, 40% fat	534	281
Mozzarella	403	236
Munster, 50% fat	230	335
Parmesan	1,290	395
Provolone	881	383
Ricotta	274	181
Roquefort	662	378
Processed cheese, 45% fat	547	282
Processed cheese, 50% fat	355	339

By comparison 100g cottage cheese contains only 95 mg calcium and 108 kcal per 100g and cream cheese 98 mg calcium and 279 kcal.

PLANT FOODS
Calcium content and energy value

	Average calcium mg/100g	Energy kcal/100g
Almonds	252	622
Brazil nuts	132	693
Broccoli	105	22
Chickpeas, dried	110	314
Chives	129	—
Dandelion leaves*	158	—
Fennel	109	—
Figs, dried	193	242
Horseradish	105	60
Kale	212	29
Mung beans, dried	123	280
Mustard greens/mustard cress	214	—
Navy/haricot beans, dried	106	301
Parsley*	245	—
Pigeon peas, dried	121	291
Pistachio nuts	136	623
Rose hips	257	91
Sesame seeds	783	562
Soybeans	257	357
Soy flour	195	370
Spinach*	126	14
Sunflower seeds	360	245
Tofu (soybean curd)	504	70
Watercress	180	—
Wheat bran	110	206

* High in oxalic acid

Vitamin D

Vitamin D promotes absorption of calcium from the gut and reabsorption of calcium by the kidneys. In most healthy people the liver contains several months' supply of vitamin D. This is derived from two sources, from foods containing vitamin D and from the action of sunlight on a cholesterol-like compound in the skin. Foods rich in vitamin D are oily fish (sardines, herring, mackerel, tuna), liver and eggs. In some countries, milk, margarine and some cereals are fortified with vitamin D. The daily dietary requirement for children and adults is 400 IU (an international unit is $\frac{1}{40}$ of a microgram) and for the elderly 800 IU. Its use in the treatment of osteoporosis is briefly discussed on page 150.

Other foods

Two other nutrients – protein and vitamin C – are also important for healthy bones. Protein is essential for the synthesis of collagen, which accounts for about a third of bone mass, and vitamin C plays an important part in collagen synthesis.

A mix of animal and plant protein is preferable to all-animal protein (high consumption of animal protein is a risk factor for osteoporosis, remember) and vegetarians should be careful to combine rice/beans, wheat/nuts, bread/lentils, etc. so that the protein they eat is "complete", containing all the essential amino acids simultaneously. Most nutritionists recommend a daily protein intake of 1g protein per kilogram (2.2 lbs) of body weight. For most people that means less than $3\frac{1}{2}$ oz (100g) or protein per day.

At present the RDAs for vitamin C are 45 mg per day for children, 60 mg per day for adults and 100 mg during pregnancy and breast-feeding. Some nutritionists believe these amounts are much too low. The best natural sources of vitamin C are kiwi fruit, blackcurrants, citrus fruit, green peppers, cauliflower, potatoes and leafy green vegetables. Being water-soluble, vitamin C is easily destroyed by cooking and canning.

WHAT DRUGS ARE USED TO TREAT OSTEOPOROSIS?

The first point to make is that ALL DRUGS MUST BE PRESCRIBED BY AN AUTHORIZED MEDICAL PRACTITIONER AND TAKEN UNDER MEDICAL SUPERVISION. Only a general outline of the various drugs used in the treatment of osteoporosis is given here.

Before prescribing medication a physician has to answer various questions. Is the patient especially at risk of osteoporosis or, alternatively, how far has the osteoporotic process progressed? Is the patient's state of health good, average or poor for her/his age? Is osteoporosis the primary disorder, or is it secondary to some other condition? What are the side effects of taking a particular medication, and are its beneficial effects likely to outweigh them? Can the medication concerned be given as a pill, or does it have to be injected or given in some other way?

In osteoporosis, the aim of medication is to subtly alter the mechanisms which control bone remodeling so that bone destruction and bone rebuilding are brought into balance. These mechanisms are still not fully understood. For an atom of calcium in a spoonful of yogurt to be absorbed through the gut, transported in the blood to a bone remodeling site, and deposited in a crystal of hydroxyapatite growing on a collagen fiber secreted by an osteoblast ... requires hundreds, if not thousands, of discrete chemical steps, many of them regulated by hormones. Hormones are therefore an obvious form of medication. Those currently used in the treatment of osteoporosis are estrogen (for women) and testosterone (for men), calcitonin and vitamin D (a hormone precursor). Calcium supplements are fairly commonly prescribed if calcium is deficient in the diet. Other forms of treatment involving fluoride therapy and a group of phosphorus compounds called biophosphonates are still regarded as experimental − their efficacy, benefits and disadvantages are still not sufficiently known. The possibility of using parathyroid hormone to stimulate bone turnover (between them, calcitonin/vitamin D and parathyroid hormone control the rate at which bone is dismantled and rebuilt) is also being investigated.

Estrogen

Although the precise way in which estrogen exerts its effect on the skeleton is not known, there is now sufficient empirical evidence for us to be able to state, unequivocally, that estrogen, taken as a drug, is effective in the prevention and treatment of osteoporosis. It may have a direct effect on bone cells, stimulating osteoblasts or inhibiting osteoclasts, or it may exert its effects by influencing the formation or action or parathyroid hormone, vitamin D or calcitonin.

The clearest evidence for a relationship between estrogen and bone status is that in women osteoporosis accelerates after the menopause. The main hormonal change at the menopause is that the ovaries cease to produce female hormones, estrogens and progestogens. Surgical removal of the ovaries before the menopause has the same effect. The menstrual cycle ceases. Temperature regulation becomes temporarily less efficient, hence the "hot flashes" or "hot flushes" which many women find such a nuisance. There may be mood changes and irritability. The tissues of the vagina become dryer and thinner. There are also slower processes at work, such as a change in the composition of fat in the blood, which increases the risk of thrombosis and coronary heart disease. In younger women, estrogen has a protective effect against cardiovascular disease. After the menopause, women begin to catch up with men in this respect.

The other slow change associated with estrogen withdrawal is accelerated loss of bone. All women are affected, but only a third go on to develop osteoporosis severe enough to cause fractures and other obvious symptoms.

Most experts now accept that estrogen is the most powerful anti-bone loss drug for women. This does not mean that every woman of menopausal or pre-menopausal age should have estrogen replacement therapy (ERT). A lack of estrogen is not the only cause of osteoporosis. If it were, osteoporotic fractures would not occur in women who take estrogen after the menopause, but they do, although they are much less common than in women who do not take estrogen. So ERT in combination with other measures such as more exercise and increased calcium intake, or calcium supplements, might be more beneficial than ERT alone. Exercise and extra calcium might also enable the dosage of estrogen to be reduced, which is desirable, since ERT is not without risks.

When taken alone, estrogen has been shown to increase the risk of cancer of the endometrium (inner lining of the uterus), although this risk can be decreased considerably by taking progesterone as well. There are also indications that long-term use of estrogen may increase the risk of breast cancer. This particular risk is not reduced by progesterone. With estrogen supplementation there is also an increased risk of venous thrombosis and pulmonary embolism, hypertension, and gallstones.

At this moment general medical opinion as far as osteoporosis is concerned is that estrogen should be given only to women who are especially at risk and to women in whom there are no contraindications, that is to women who do not have cardiovascular problems, etc. The consensus is that the greatest benefit is gained by starting ERT shortly after the menopause and tailing it off after 10 years or so. Administration is by tablets or by implants under the skin. The value of ERT for women with established osteoporosis 15 or more years after the menopause is not yet proven.

Calcitonin

Calcitonin, a hormone secreted by the thyroid gland, is thought to slow down bone loss by discouraging oesteoclast activity. Its other action is to stimulate reabsorption of calcium and phosphates by the kidneys, preventing excessive losses of these in the urine. These complementary effects are enhanced when calcitonin is given as a medication.

Calcitonin is sometimes prescribed as an alternative to ERT, if ERT is declined or contraindicated. However, it is not widely used. It is expensive, and at the moment has to be given by daily injections, although a nasal spray is currently being tested. The more fundamental reason for its limited use is that it ceases to have a positive effect after about a year or a year and a half.

Vitamin D

In the sense that vitamin D is made by the body itself, secreted directly into the bloodstream, and transported to distant sites where it has a specific effect, it can be regarded as a hormone. However, the form of vitamin D made in the skin in response to short-wave ultraviolet light and the vitamin D present in food are inactive. They are converted to a partially active form in the liver and into a final active form in the kidneys.

Vitamin D affects bone turnover by enabling calcium to be absorbed from the gut and reabsorbed by the kidneys. However, when vitamin D levels in the blood rise above a certain level, bones start to *lose* their calcium. Irradiation of the skin does not lead to vitamin D toxicity, but oral supplementation can. Vitamin D supplementation may be essential if exposure to sunlight is difficult or the diet is deficient, or if the kidneys are unable to convert the vitamin to its final form.

Calcium supplements

For people who cannot or do not eat enough calcium-containing foods to satisfy their daily calcium requirement (see page 140), calcium supplements are the obvious solution. Some people cannot eat dairy foods because the lactose in them causes bloating and diarrhea. Others are concerned about the high calorie value of many dairy foods. Others simply do not like their taste.

Although calcium tablets can be bought over the counter, they are best prescribed or bought on the recommendation of a doctor as it is not always clear what the elemental calcium content of each tablet is nor its availability. Some calcium preparations include vitamin D. Calcium citrate is often prescribed for people who secrete little stomach acid, without which calcium cannot be absorbed.

People receiving calcium supplementation are encouraged to drink plenty of water to maintain a high urine volume. Kidney stones are a contraindication for calcium supplementation.

Sodium fluoride   In the normal diet, consumption of fluoride is extremely small, less than 0.5 mg per day, most of it derived from the fluoride added to drinking water or from fish such as sardines and mackerel. Nevertheless fluoride is essential for healthy teeth and bones because it increases the stability of their mineral content. At larger doses it also stimulates osteoblasts to form new collagen, predominantly in trabecular bone. But in very large doses, or when the amount which accumulates in bone is too high, its effect on bone quality may be negative.

Although sodium fluoride tablets have been prescribed for osteoporosis for more than 20 years, their efficacy and safety is still being assessed. There is evidence that fluoride therapy, accompanied by an adequate intake of calcium and vitamin D, reduces susceptibility to compression fractures of the vertebrae.

Wallbars Hanging onto furniture, doors and other household objects is dangerous. In most cases there are partnered exercises which exert traction in almost the same way, so please choose these rather than put yourself at risk.

The best solution would be to install your private set of wall bars. The sketch opposite shows the simplest and sturdiest method of construction – wooden uprights which reach from floor to ceiling and wooden bars which slot through them at both sides. The uprights should be firmly secured to the floor (without carpet beneath) and ceiling, and also to the wall (a solid wall, not a flimsy partition wall) at several points. The bars should be not less than 35mm/1⅜ inch in diameter and the uprights need to be of similar thickness. Ideally the bars should be about 75cm/30 inches long and set at least 10cm/4 inches from the wall; that means that the uprights need to be about 18cm/7 inches wide. The bars are glued fast into their slots.

A compromise solution would be to adapt a doorway to take bars, provided the door frame is good and sturdy. Various brackets and supports can be used to take the ends of the bars, but they must be very firmly fixed. Remember, the bars have to take all or most of your weight.

Another solution would be to buy a ladder – wood or lightweight metal, provided it has rungs rather than steps – and attach it to the wall. The ideal would be a ladder which stretched from floor to ceiling, so that it could be fixed to both for extra security.

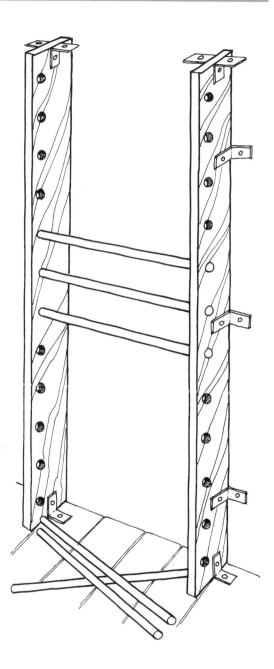

wallbars

REFERENCES

Introduction

J F Fries. Aging, illness, and health policy: implications of the compression of morbidity. *Perspectives in Biology and Medicine*, 31: 407–428, 1988.

B L Riggs and L J Melton III (editors). *Osteoporosis – etiology, diagnosis and management.* Raven Press, New York, 1988.

N B Watts. Osteoporosis. *American Family Physician*, 38/5: 193–207, 1988.

N M Resnick and S L Greenspan. 'Senile' osteoporosis reconsidered. *Journal of the American Medical Association*, 261: 1025–1029, 1989.

What is osteoporosis?

M Motelovitz (editor). Climacteric and Osteoporosis. *Clinical Obstetrics and Gynecology*, 30: 787–884, 1987.

N B Watts. Osteoporosis. *American Family Physician*, 38: 193–207, 1988.

F S Kaplan. Osteoporosis: Pathophysiology and Prevention. Ciba-Geigy Clinical Symposia, 39: 1, 1987.

Who is at risk?

J F Aloia et al. Risk factors for postmenopausal osteoporosis. *The American Journal of Medicine*, 78: 95–100, 1985.

S Y Lam et al. Gynaecological disorders and risk factors in premenopausal women predisposing to osteoporosis – a review. *British Journal of Obstetrics and Gynaecology*, 95: 963–972, 1988.

E Seeman et al. Reduced bone mass in daughters of women with osteoporosis. *The New England Journal of Medicine*, 320: 554–558, 1989.

How is bone gained and lost?

W A Peck and W L Woods. The cells of bone, in *Osteoporosis, etiology, diagnosis and management*, edited by B L Riggs and L J Melton III, pp. 1–44, Raven Press, New York, 1988.

A M Parfitt. Bone remodelling, in *Osteoporosis, etiology, diagnosis and management*, edited by B L Riggs and L J Melton III, pp. 45–93, Raven Press, New York, 1988.

How is bone loss measured?

B Murby and I Fogelman. Bone mineral measurement in clinical practice. *British Journal of Hospital Medicine*, 453–458, 1987.

F M Hall et al. Bone mineral screening for osteoporosis. *The New England Journal of Medicine*, 316, 212–214, 1987.

D J Sartoris and D Resnick. Osteoporosis: update on densitometric techniques. *The Journal of Musculoskeletal Medicine*, 6, 108–123, 1989.

Effects of mechanical stimuli on bone remodeling

L E Lanyon. Functional strain as determinant of bone remodelling. *Calcified Tissue International*, 36: S56–S61, 1984.

S C Cowin. Mechanical modelling of the stress adaptation process in bone. *Calcified Tissue International*, 36: S98–S103, 1984.

L E Lanyon. Functional strain in bone tissue as an objective, and controlling stimulus for adaptive bone remodelling. *Journal of Biomechanics*, 20: 1083–1093, 1987.

D R Carter. Mechanical loading history and skeletal biology. *Journal of Biomechanics*, 20: 1095–1109, 1987.

H M Frost. Vital biomechanics: proposed general concepts for skeletal adaptation to mechanical usage. *Calcified Tissue International*, 42: 145–156, 1988.

R T Whalen et al. Influence of physical activity on the regulation of bone density. *Journal of Biomechanics*, 21: 825–837, 1988.

Effects of mechanical stimuli on human bone

K A Larson et al. Decreasing the incidence of osteoporosis-related injuries through diet and exercise. *Public Health Reports*, 99: 609–613, 1984.

N A Pocock et al. Physical fitness as a major determinant of femoral neck and lumbar spine bone mineral density. *Journal of Clinical Investigation*, 78: 618–621, 1986.

D A Bailey et al. Physical activity, nutrition, bone density and osteoporosis. *Australian Journal of Science and Medicine in Sport*, 18: 3–8, 1986.

A Simkin et al. Increased trabecular bone density due to bone-loading exercises in postmenopausal osteoporotic women. *Calcified Tissue International*, 40: 59–63, 1987.

J Ayalon et al. Dynamic bone-loading exercises for postmenopausal osteoporotic women: effect on the density of the distal radius. *Archives of Physical Medicine and Rehabilitation*, 68: 280–283, 1987.

R Chow et al. Effect of two randomised exercise programmes on bone mass of healthy postmenopausal women. *British Medical Journal*, 295: 1441–1444, 1987.

E L Smith et al. Effects of inactivity and exercise on bone. *The Physician and Sports Medicine*, 15, 91–100, 1987.

J E Block et al. Does exercise prevent osteoporosis? *Journal of the American Medical Association*, 257, 3115–3117, 1987.

E S Orwoll et al. The effect of swimming exercises on bone mineral contents. *Clinical Research*, 35, 194A, 1987.

D Schapira. Physical exercise in the prevention and treatment of osteoporosis – a review. *Journal of the Royal Society of Medicine*, 81: 461–463, 1988.

G A Dalski et al. Weight-bearing exercise training and lumbar bone mineral content in postmenopausal women. *Annals of Internal Medicine*, 108: 824–828, 1988.

M C Beverly et al. Local bone mineral response to brief exercise that stresses the skeleton. *British Medical Journal*, 299: 233–235, 1989.

E L Smith et al. Deterring bone loss by exercise intervention in premenopausal and postmenopausal women. *Calcified Tissue International*, 44: 312–321, 1989.

L A Colleti et al. The effects of muscle-building exercises on bone mineral density of the radius, spine and hip in young men. *Calcified Tissue International*, 45: 12–14, 1989.

E L Smith and C Gilligan. Mechanical forces and bone (a review), in *Bone and Mineral Research*, edited by W A Peck, pp. 139–173, Elsevier, Amsterdam, 1989.

I Leichter, A Simkin et al. Gain in mass density of bone following strenuous physical activity. *Journal of Orthopaedic Research*, 7: 86–90, 1989.

Effects of diet on bone status

R Marcus: Calcium intake and skeletal integrity: is there a critical relationship? *Journal of Nutrition*, 117: 631–635, 1986.

B Riis et al. Does calcium supplementation prevent postmenopausal bone loss? *New England Journal of Medicine*, 316: 173–177, 1987.

F A Tylavsky et al. Dietary factors in bone health of elderly lacto-ovovegetarian and omnivorous women. *American Journal of Clinical Nutrition*, 48: 842–849, 1988.

A G Marsh et al. Vegetarian lifestyle and bone mineral density. *American Journal of Clinical Nutrition*, 48: 837–841, 1988.

J A Kanis et al. Calcium supplementation of the diet – not justified by present evidence. *British Medical Journal*, 298: 205–208, 1989.

E Barret-Connor. The Recommended Dietary Allowances for Calcium in the Elderly: too little, too late. *Calcified Tissue International*, 44: 303–307, 1989.

H Scherz, G Kloos and F Senser, editors. *Food Composition and Nutrition Tables*. Published for Deutsche Forschunganstalt für Lebensmittelchemie by Wissenschaftliche Verlagsgesellschaft mbH, Stuttgart, 1986.

Drug therapy for osteoporosis

J S Gallagher. Drug therapy of osteoporosis: Calcium, estrogen and vitamin D, in B L Riggs and L J Melton, (editors): *Osteoporosis – Etiology, Diagnosis and Management*, Raven Press, New York, 1988.

C H Chestnut. Drug therapy: Calcitonin, Biphosphonates, Anabolic Steroids and hPTH (1–34). Ibid. pp. 403–414.

E F Eriksen, S F Hodgson and B L Riggs. Treatment of Osteoporosis with Sodium Fluoride. Ibid. pp 415–432.

Consensus Development Conference: Prophylaxis and treatment of osteoporosis. *British Medical Journal*, 295: 914–915, 1987.

U Barzel. Estrogen in the prevention and treatment of postmenopausal osteoporosis: a review. *American Journal of Medicine*, 85: 847–850, 1988.

references

INDEX

PICTURE CREDITS

The publishers extend their thanks and appreciation to Albi Zarfati for taking all the exercise photographs, and to Ora Chayoun and Boaz Rodansky for so cheerfully and tirelessly posing for them.

The artwork on pages 117, 126, 135, 137, 139 and 152 is by Jane Cope. The illustrations on page 118 are by Frank H. Netter MD, and are reproduced from Clinical Symposia 39/1 'Osteoporosis: Pathology and Prevention', courtesy of CIBA-Geigy Ltd, Basle, Switzerland, and the photographs on pages 127 are from *Sandorama* 1987/IV, reproduced by kind permission of Sandoz Ltd, Basle, Switzerland.

The single and dual photo absorptiometry photographs on pages 129 and 130 are reproduced by courtesy of the Jerusalem Osteoporosis Center, and the photograph of Compton spectometry testing on page 132 by courtesy of the Hadassah University Hospital, Jerusalem, and the Jerusalem Osteoporosis Center.